THE TRUTH ABOUT ALCOHOL

THE TRUTH ABOUT ALCOHOL

MARK J. KITTLESON, PH.D.
Southern Illinois University
General Editor

WILLIAM KANE, PH.D.
University of New Mexico
Adviser

RICHELLE RENNEGARBE, PH.D.
McKendree College
Adviser

Barry Youngerman
Principal Author

☑®
Facts On File, Inc.

The Truth About Alcohol

Written and Developed by BOOK BUILDERS LLC

Facts On File, Inc.
132 West 31st Street
New York NY 10001

Library of Congress Cataloging-in-Publication Data

The truth about alcohol / Mark J. Kittleson, general editor; William Kane, adviser; Richelle Rennegarbe, adviser; Barry Youngerman, principal author.
  p. cm.
 Includes index
 ISBN 0-8160-5298-0 (hc: alk. paper)
 1. Teenagers—Alcohol use. 2. Alcoholism—Prevention. I. Youngerman, Barry. II. Kittleson, Mark J., 1952–
 RJ506.D78F33 2004
 362.292′0835—dc22

                                                          2004000509

Facts On File books are available at special discounts when purchased in bulk quantities for businesses, associations, institutions, or sales promotions. Please call our Special Sales Department in New York at (212) 967-8800 or (800) 322-8755.

You can find Facts On File on the World Wide Web at http://www.factsonfile.com

Text design by David Strelecky
Cover design by Cathy Rincon
Graphs by Sholto Ainslie, Patricia Meschino

Printed in the United States of America

MP Hermitage 10 9 8 7 6 5 4 3 2 1

This book is printed on acid-free paper.

CONTENTS

LIST OF ILLUSTRATIONS

PREFACE

In developing this series, The Truth About, we have taken time to review some of the most pressing problems facing our youth today. Issues such as alcohol and drug abuse, depression, family problems, sexual activity, and eating disorders are at the top of a list of growing concerns. It is the intent of these books to provide vital facts while also dispelling myths about these terribly important and all-too-common situations. These are authoritative resources that kids can turn to in order to get an accurate answer to a specific question or to research the history of a problem, giving them access to the most current related data available. It is also a reference for parents, teachers, counselors, and others who work with youth and require detailed information.

Let's take a brief look at the issues associated with each of those topics. Alcohol and drug use and abuse continue to be a national concern. Today's young people often use drugs to escape the extraordinary pressures of today. In doing so they are losing their ability to learn how to cope effectively. Without the internal resources to cope with pressure, adolescents turn increasingly back to addictive behaviors. As a result, the problems and solutions are interrelated. Also, the speed with which the family structure is changing often leaves kids with no outlet for stress and no access to support mechanisms.

In addition, a world of youth faces the toughest years of their lives, dealing with the strong physiological urges that accompany sexual desire. Only when young people are presented the facts honestly, without indoctrination, are they likely to connect risk taking with certain behaviors. This reference set relies on knowledge as the most important tool in research and education.

Finally, one of the most puzzling issues of our times is that of eating disorders. Paradoxically, while our youth are obsessed with thinness and beauty, and go to extremes to try to meet perceived societal expectations, they are also increasingly plagued by obesity. Here too separating the facts from fiction is an important tool in research and learning.

As much as possible, this series presents the facts through honest discussions and reports of the most up-to-date research. Knowing the facts associated with health-related questions and problems will help young people make informed decisions in school and throughout life.

Mark J. Kittleson
General Editor

HOW TO
USE THIS BOOK

NOTE TO STUDENTS

Knowledge is power. By possessing knowledge you have the ability to make decisions, ask follow-up questions, or know where to go to obtain more information. In the world of health that is power! That is the purpose of this book—to provide you the power you need to obtain unbiased, accurate information and *The Truth About Alcohol.*

Topics in each volume of The Truth About are arranged in alphabetical order, from A to Z. Each of these entries defines its topic and explains in detail the particular issue. At the end of most entries are cross-references to related topics. A list of all topics by letter can be found in the table of contents or at the back of the book in the index.

How have these books been compiled? First, the publisher worked with me to identify some of the country's leading authorities on key issues in health education. These individuals were asked to identify some of the major concerns that young people have about such topics. The writers read the literature, spoke with health experts, and incorporated their own life and professional experiences to pull together the most up-to-date information on health issues, particularly those of interest to adolescents and of concern in Healthy People 2010.

Throughout the alphabetical entries, the reader will find sidebars that separate fact from fiction. There are question-and-answer boxes that attempt to address the most common questions that youth ask about sensitive topics. In addition, readers will find a special feature called "Teens Speak"—case studies of teens with personal stories related to the topic in hand.

This may be one of the most important books you will ever read. Please share it with your friends, families, teachers, and classmates. Remember, you possess the power to control your future. One way to affect your course is through the acquisition of knowledge. Good luck and keep healthy.

NOTE TO LIBRARIANS

This book, along with the rest of the series, The Truth About, serves as a wonderful resource for young researchers. It contains a variety of facts, case studies, and further readings that the reader can use to help answer questions, formulate new questions, or determine where to go to find more information. Even though the topics may be considered delicate by some, do not be afraid to ask patrons if they have questions. Feel free to direct them to the appropriate sources, but do not press them if you encounter reluctance. The best we can do as educators is to let young people know that we are there when they need us.

Mark J. Kittleson, Ph.D.
General Editor

ADDICTIVE BEHAVIORS AND ALCOHOL

In common speech, the term *heavy drinking* can be very vague. However, according to the National Institute of Alcohol Abuse and Alcoholism, a heavy drinker consumes five or more drinks (or sometimes four, for a woman) on at least five different occasions during a month. In other words, anyone who drinks a six-pack of beer once or twice every weekend is considered a heavy drinker.

Some adults can be heavy drinkers for years without falling into the category of alcohol abusers, people who consume alcohol excessively. They may always drink in a pleasant social setting, never drive after drinking, and be responsible spouses, parents, and employees. For young people, however, heavy drinking is usually very difficult to manage and is generally associated with abuse.

The different impact that alcohol has on different individuals makes it difficult to generalize when discussing alcohol use, abuse, and addiction: What affects one person one way may affect someone else differently. Still, by definition, alcohol abuse is always a problem behavior. The National Institute of Alcohol Abuse and Alcoholism defines the term as "a pattern of drinking that results in one or more of the following situations within a 12-month period:

- Failure to fulfill major work, school, or home responsibilities;
- Drinking in situations that are physically dangerous, such as while driving a car or operating machinery;
- Having recurring alcohol-related legal problems, such as being arrested for driving under the influence of alcohol or for physically hurting someone while drunk; and

1

■ Continued drinking despite having ongoing relationship problems that are caused or worsened by the drinking."

A person can abuse alcohol without being an **alcoholic**, that is, without the physical dependence. The cravings may not be overpowering, and the person may be able to stop drinking on any one occasion. However, the abusive behavior patterns are difficult to overcome, and it may be difficult for alcohol abusers to develop safe drinking behaviors.

DEFINITIONS OF DRINKING BEHAVIORS

The terms *alcohol* **addiction,** *alcohol dependency,* and *alcoholism* are often used to mean the same thing. However, they can be used to highlight different aspects of the same behavior.

The term addiction can be used for any drug, as well as for other patterns of behavior such as gambling. Addiction is a chronic disease in which a person has a physical and psychological need or craving for the substance or behavior. It lasts for a long period of time and is difficult or impossible to cure. It can be controlled, but relapses are common, in which the person slips back into his or her old, problematic behavior.

Binge drinking refers to a period of drinking five or more drinks at one sitting; this is sometimes called heavy episodic drinking—"episodic" because it only happens now and then. Some reports consider a woman to be engaged in binge drinking if she drinks *four* or more drinks at one time.

Dependency is used only for drug-related addictions. It usually refers to a physical condition in the addict's brain and other organs. Anyone who is dependent on a drug needs periodic doses of the drug just to avoid painful, uncomfortable, or frightening symptoms. Those symptoms are summed up in the term **withdrawal**, which is discussed later in this section.

Alcoholism means an addiction to alcohol. It includes a strong craving or compulsion to drink at regular intervals (every day, for many alcoholics, or just periodically, for example, on weekends, for others). It includes a loss of control; once an alcoholic takes one drink, he or she generally cannot stop. Alcoholics also have a physical dependence on the drug and experience withdrawal symptoms if they stop drinking.

Some alcoholics vary their behaviors between episodes of excessive drinking and periods of sobriety. Alcoholics who have overcome their cravings and have been sober for a long period of time are usually considered "alcoholics in recovery."

Tolerance

People who drink a large amount of alcohol, especially those who have become dependent on alcohol, usually develop a degree of **tolerance**. People who need to drink more to get the same mental effect, or who get less of a buzz when they drink their usual amount, probably have an acquired tolerance to alcohol. They say things like, "I really can hold my liquor," or "I can drink you under the table."

Tolerance occurs as the brain and nervous system become accustomed to alcohol. The nerve cells adapt their normal functioning to compensate for the effects of the drug. However, even in the brain, the tolerance can only go so far. A heavy drinker may need more alcohol to get drunk but only a little bit more to black out, go into a coma, or die. Also, as tolerance develops and drinkers continually increase their dose, the brain may adjust but other organs can be seriously damaged.

An alcoholic's liver can develop **metabolic tolerance** to alcohol by learning to break down or metabolize a larger amount of the substance in a given period of time than the liver of a nonalcoholic. However, none of the other vital organs are so flexible. A given amount of alcohol inflicts the same amount of damage to an alcoholic's stomach, heart, arteries, bone, and other organs as it does with a casual drinker, even if the alcoholic never feels drunk.

A high degree of tolerance can give heavy drinkers a false sense of security. They may not feel drunk, but in all likelihood their coordination, reflexes, and judgment are impaired. People who develop a high tolerance to alcohol should not be fooled into thinking that they can safely drive or perform other difficult or dangerous tasks just because they don't feel drunk.

Tolerance may vary with the environment. Some people can drive home along a familiar route even after a couple of drinks. But if they try a different route, the same level of blood alcohol can cause much greater impairment.

Alcoholics often lose their high level of tolerance after an extended period of time, and then even one drink makes them drunk. This may be a sign of liver damage and should not be ignored. It also can lead to severe, unexpected intoxication, which is especially dangerous when driving.

Withdrawal

When alcoholics or heavy drinkers suddenly stop drinking, or when they drastically cut back on the amount they drink, they usually experience some form of withdrawal. Withdrawal refers to the combination of painful and uncomfortable symptoms they feel as their bodies try to re-adapt to an alcohol-free bloodstream.

When the brain and nervous system are suddenly deprived of alcohol, they quickly try to readjust to their normal, drug-free behavior. This sounds simple, but it is very unpleasant to experience. According to scientists, the nerve cells in the brain become accustomed to working extra hard to overcome the depressing effects of alcohol. For a while, they continue to work overtime, but without alcohol to slow them down, they are in a super-excited state.

A few hours after the last drink, the patient may feel weak, shaky, and anxious, and usually suffers from headache, nausea, and stomach cramps. Somewhat later, he or she begins to feel agitated and starts to crave another drink. As the hours go by, severe **tremors**, or shaking, may develop, followed by **hallucinations**—seeing and hearing things that aren't there.

In more severe cases, brain seizures may occur, and need to be treated immediately with powerful drugs. The worst-case scenario is called **delirium tremens**, or the D.T.'s. These intense, terrifying hallucinations continue for three to four days, accompanied by high fevers and extremely aggressive behavior. A century ago, up to 40 percent of D.T. cases resulted in death; improvements in treatment have reduced the rate to 5 percent, according to a 1998 study reported in the *Southern Medical Journal*.

The majority of cases of severe withdrawal occur in older people who have been drinking for years. But people as young as 20 also can experience withdrawal, depending on how much and how long they have been drinking.

Teens should also bear in mind that even a mild withdrawal could set the stage for more severe problems later on, due to the **kindling effect**, which means that when alcoholics go through withdrawal more than once, the symptoms often get more severe each time. The nerve cells seem to become kindled—they are not charged up enough to cause problems now but any additional charge in the future could push them over the top. Evidence suggests that people who show this effect are in greater danger of relapse (returning to alcohol abuse) and also are more likely to suffer brain damage.

Even relatively mild cases of withdrawal may need medical attention. Anyone who makes the courageous decision to fight alcohol dependency should arrange to have help in advance.

WHAT ARE THE SYMPTOMS AND BEHAVIORS OF ALCOHOL ABUSE AND ALCOHOLISM?

Teenagers are among alcohol's most obvious victims. When young people drink, lots of bad things often happen—to the drinkers and to those around them. As a result, Congress and state legislators have made it illegal to sell or serve alcohol in the United States to people under 21 years old. However, the laws have not been easy to enforce, and underage drinking continues.

In fact, many kids have fallen into dangerous habits of heavy drinking, abuse, and even addiction. Other kids are at risk of doing the same; many of them may not even be aware of the dangers they face.

In the 22 articles that follow on the problems associated with alcohol and addiction, you can read about the main types of harmful alcohol-related behavior and learn how common they are among young people. You also can discover information on the risk factors for alcohol abuse, and the signs that show whether you or someone you know has begun to develop addictive problems with alcohol. This information may help keep you out of harm's way, or help you start dealing with any problems you may already have.

The signs of alcohol abuse

Some alcoholics are so skilled at concealing their problem that even friends, family members, or coworkers may not suspect the extent of their drinking. In the majority of cases, however, especially with younger drinkers, some signs of alcohol abuse can be a tip-off to concerned loved ones. Here are some of them:

- Drinking alone
- Being unable to cut back
- Drinking in the morning
- Keeping a supply of alcohol in a hidden place
- Wishing they had a drink
- Going to school or work drunk
- Drinking even while taking prescription drugs, against the doctor's orders

- Gulping instead of sipping alcohol
- Lying to family and friends about drinking
- Finding excuses to drink
- Drinking more than they intended
- Saying it's just a phase
- Drinking to escape problems, or to fall asleep
- Having blackouts
- Spending large amounts of time sleeping off hangovers
- Losing interest in schoolwork and starting to fall behind
- Avoiding friends who don't drink
- Feeling tired all the time without being ill
- Feeling more irritable than usual
- Getting angry if someone raises the subject of your drinking

The stages of drinking problems

Every human being possesses his or her own physical, psychological, and social makeup. Among people who drink alcohol, not everyone develops exactly the same habits. Still, many people who become alcoholics do seem to follow a particular pattern. This is known as **progression**, or moving from one stage to another, more serious stage.

There are different definitions of the stages. The National Council on Alcoholism and Drug Dependence states, "The typical progression from alcohol use to addiction involves the following stages:

- Experimental stage: curiosity about the effects of alcohol causes the user to try alcohol one or more times;
- Social stage: alcohol is used occasionally in social situations such as parties or with friends;
- Dependent stage: the user becomes obsessed with alcohol and consumes it regularly, often alone; and
- Chronic stage: the user feels constant emotional or physical pain, which can be lessened only by alcohol."

ADDICTING SUBSTANCES AMONG TEENS: WHERE DOES ALCOHOL RANK?

Despite all the attention that marijuana, cocaine, club drugs, and other illegal substances get in the media, alcohol remains the most widely used—and abused—addicting drug among young Americans, even including tobacco. The 2002 Monitoring the Future Survey of the National Institute on Drug Abuse found that nearly twice as many eighth, 10th, and 12th graders had consumed alcohol in the previous month than had smoked cigarettes (48, 35, and 20 percent compared with 26, 18, and 11 percent).

Experts may debate whether one particular drug is more or less addictive than another; that is, whether a user would find it harder to give up alcohol or, for example, marijuana. That fact is hard to determine, but the number of teenagers who suffer from alcohol abuse dwarfs the numbers for any other drug—showing that alcohol use is a serious problem.

The latest figures, according to the National Household Survey on Drug Abuse (NHSDA), a project of the federal Department of Health and Human Services that gets its information from families themselves, reported that in 2000, 2.6 percent of all kids aged 12–17 were heavy drinkers. According to the NHSDA, a heavy drinker had "five or more drinks on the same occasion at least five different days in the past 30 days." In addition, another 7.8 percent were binge drinkers, who had five or more drinks at least once but fewer than five times in that same 30-day period.

This adds up to a large number of young people—more than five million teenage alcohol abusers, according to the National Institute on Alcohol Abuse and Alcoholism (NIAAA). Of course, not all of these kids are addicted. Hopefully, most of the bingers will avoid becoming addicted. In 1996, according to the Substance Abuse and Mental Health Services Administration (SAMHSA), 182,000 adolescents or young adults under age 20 received treatment for substance abuse in the United States, and 55 percent of them were treated for abusing alcohol (either alone or with other substances).

Compare those facts to other drugs. Each year, Monitoring the Future, a project under the U.S. Department of Health and Human Services, surveys about 50,000 kids in grades 8, 10, and 12 about their use of drugs, including alcohol and tobacco. The good news is that nearly every drug, including alcohol, saw small but significant declines in use in the past few years. But the pattern remains the same—alcohol is abused more than any other drug. In fact, alcohol is abused more than all illicit drugs combined, including marijuana, cocaine, inhalants, hallucinogens (such as LSD), ecstasy, heroin, **amphetamines**, barbiturates, and tranquilizers.

For example, in 2002, Monitoring the Future found that, among 12th graders, 48.6 percent had used alcohol at least once and 30.3 percent had gotten drunk in the previous 30 days, as compared with 25.4 percent who used *all other drugs*. Over the course of the year, 71.5 percent had used alcohol, 50.4 percent had gotten drunk, and 41.0 percent had used other drugs.

WHAT ARE THE RISK FACTORS?

A number of **risk factors**, or causes, may influence a teen who has experimented with alcohol to lose control and become dependent. Some of these causes, such as family history and friends' behavior, are beyond the person's control. However, there is always *something* a person can do to limit the impact of these factors and prevent them from running his or her life.

Family history

Perhaps the greatest single risk factor for alcohol abuse is a family history of alcoholism. People have long noticed that alcohol abuse runs in families, but they didn't know how it was passed along from one generation to the next. Was it a behavior pattern that children learned from watching their parents, or was it some inherited chemical factor that made certain people more susceptible to the dangers of alcohol? Or was it some combination of both factors?

By now, the majority of scientists who have studied the subject believe that the family's genes are responsible for alcoholism in families. Studies of identical twins have found that if one twin is alcoholic, the other is quite likely to be alcoholic too. Other studies have found that kids from alcoholic families tend to have alcohol problems even if adopted and raised by nonalcoholics—and vice-versa.

Take note that the *majority* of children from families with a history of alcoholism do *not* themselves become alcoholic. However, more of them do than children of nonalcoholic families. According to alcohol researcher D. W. Goodwin, 20 to 25 percent of sons and brothers of alcoholics, and 5 percent of daughters and sisters of alcoholics, become alcoholics themselves. Also, these kids tend to become alcohol abusers and alcoholics at an earlier age than other people, and may suffer a more severe form of the disease.

Friends who drink

Most people are influenced by their friends, for better or worse. Unfortunately, this goes for alcohol abuse as well. If your circle of friends drinks, you may find it difficult to resist. Even if you don't become dependent, drinking among groups of teenagers often takes abusive forms.

You may believe you are strong enough to resist the influence of your friends. However, if you feel you are at risk for alcohol problems, due to family background or other factors, you may want to make a point of staying away from a circle of friends who drink.

Home and school

Problems at home and at school can sometimes lead to alcohol abuse. Most people do not try to escape their problems with drugs, but some do take that path. Alcohol, like many other drugs, may seem to help "get your mind off" your troubles. If your family is going through a rough period, such as an impending divorce; if your schoolwork has not been up to potential lately; or if you have broken up with a boyfriend or girlfriend, you may be tempted to escape your worries about these problems. This behavior can put you at risk for substance abuse.

The real danger is that you may come to think that alcohol is the only way to relieve your feelings of sadness or anxiety. If you feel that way, you are at very high risk of becoming dependent.

At times like these, becoming aware of your behaviors is even more important. Try to find healthy alternatives, such as sports or community service, to give yourself a little perspective. Always bear in mind that whatever your other problems may be, they will not be helped by adding alcohol to the situation.

Psychological factors

Kids with emotional problems are also at greater risk for alcohol abuse—just as troubled adults are. People who suffer from long-term depression are considered to be at risk; so are people who have difficulty coping with the normal problems and challenges of teen life.

For example, teens who feel insecure about their looks or social skills may turn to alcohol in the belief that getting drunk will help them overcome their shyness or inhibition. Other kids, who feel too much pressure to achieve, for example from parents, teachers, or coaches, might try to relieve the pressure by turning to alcohol.

Not every teenage alcoholic started out as an emotionally troubled kid. Some drink as a way to feel independent or to stand up to authority. Although most people will not progress from the rebellious stage to alcoholism, if someone is at risk due to other factors, she or he should probably try to find more appropriate ways of acting grown up. Some teenagers say frankly that they drink because they choose to get drunk. You can't fault their honesty, but you can ask them a simple question: If they get drunk on a regular basis, are they really in control of their behavior?

Age of onset

Researchers have found that the younger a child is when he or she begins to drink, the more likely he or she is to become dependent on alcohol. Very few of these young kids expect to become addicted.

Not all kids who take their first drink at a very early age become dependent on alcohol, but there does seem to be a pattern, as indicated in two different surveys done at a 10-year interval. A 1991 report by the American Academy of Pediatrics found that one out of seven fourth graders (who are mostly nine years old) had already become drunk at least once. Ten years later, the National Household Survey found that one out of seven of the same age cohort, who were now 19 years old, were heavy drinkers.

Given their smaller size, children absorb alcohol into their bloodstream at a faster rate than older kids or adults. They become drunk sooner and remain drunk for a longer period of time. The toxic effects on the young nervous system, which is still developing, are likely to be more serious too. These drinkers may easily become physically tolerant, or addicted, to alcohol.

The circumstances of a child's or teen's first alcohol experiences are also very important in determining how they behave in the future. In many foreign countries and among many immigrant communities in the United States, parents allow children, or even encourage them, to taste beer, wine, or even liquor at social or religious occasions. For years, researchers found lower levels of alcoholism among the children of first- or second-generation Americans with Italian, Greek, Chinese, and Jewish origins, who generally follow those traditions. Important family milestones were celebrated with a round of drinks and toasts.

For many Catholics and Jews, drinking wine plays an important role in religious ceremonies. For example, wine is usually served at the Passover seder in Jewish homes and at Christmas dinner among Italians, and kids are allowed to partake. For such kids, the researchers believe, alcohol is not a "forbidden fruit" associated with rebellion, but just another part of the traditional diet.

Experts can argue about whether such practices, if adopted in the future by all Americans, would reduce alcoholism. However, in today's world, very young drinkers usually have their first drink outside the home, which exposes them to a high level of risk.

REHABILITATION PROGRAMS

If these signs helped you realize that someone you know—perhaps yourself—has a problem with alcohol, do not despair. Although there is still much that doctors and treatment professionals do not know, many options are available to people who want to deal with their alcohol abuse.

They might first want to read the entries in this book on *Self-Help Programs* and *Recovery and Treatment*. Then they should turn to family and friends for guidance and moral support, if they feel they can. They also may need help from an organized treatment program. Many programs are available, so they may even need help in selecting which program in their area is best for them. For information on these options, please see *Hotlines and Help Sites* at the end of this book.

Teens who are fighting an addiction to alcohol may have special issues in trying to rebuild their lives. But they may have certain advantages too.

Compared to the family members of adult alcoholics, families of recovering teenagers may be more able and willing to forgive their teen for the destructive behavior of the past. After all, giving support is part of what it means to be a parent. However, many parents lose patience, and may eventually "wash their hands" of their alcoholic children, if the kids don't make a major effort to do their part in recovery.

Teachers and school staff are more likely to give the recovering alcoholic another chance, compared to employers, who may have suffered financial loss from an alcoholic employee. Finally, teenagers who have overcome alcohol addiction still have long lives ahead of them. True, no one can give them back the time they wasted, but with work and determination, they can look forward to experiencing the challenges of adult life with the wisdom and strength that recovery can sometimes give.

RISKY BUSINESS SELF-TEST

Most people in the early stages of alcohol dependence are blissfully unaware that they have a problem, or they may be trying hard not to admit it to themselves. If you drink more than once in a while, you might want to ask yourself the following 20 questions. On a piece of paper, keep a record of your answers—"yes" or "no."

Personality changes
Although other causes may account for these issues, alcohol might well be one.

- Am I losing interest in schoolwork and starting to fall behind?
- Do I avoid my old friends who don't drink?
- Do I feel tired all the time, without being ill?
- Do I feel more irritable than in the past?
- Do I get angry if someone asks me any of the questions above?
- Do I get angry if someone raises the subject of my drinking alcohol?
- Do I find myself lying to family and friends about how often and how much I drink?

Changes in drinking patterns
These are usually signs of alcohol abuse.

- Do I drink alone?
- Do I drink in the morning?
- Do I go to school or work drunk?
- Do I drink even while taking prescription drugs, against doctor's orders?
- Do I drink to escape problems, or to fall asleep?
- Do I explain my drinking as "just a phase"?
- Do I gulp instead of sip alcohol?
- Do I have blackouts, forgetting what happened while I was drinking?
- Do I spend a lot of time sleeping off hangovers?

Cravings and loss of control
These are signs that abuse may be turning into addiction:

- Do I wind up drinking more than I intended when I picked up the first glass?

- Do I keep a supply of alcohol in a hidden place?
- Do I find myself wishing I had a drink?
- Do I look for excuses to drink?

When counting up all of your answers, did you answer "yes" to more than 15 questions? If so, you should talk with someone about your drinking behaviors. (Remember, a drinking buddy is not a good choice here, unless he or she also is asking serious questions.) If *any* of the behaviors in the last two groups looks familiar to you, you should seek help.

If you still are not sure you or someone you care about has a problem, here's another question to ask yourself: Did any of the following sentences pop into your head as you read the list above? These are things that alcoholics in denial tend to say:

- I'll never become an alcoholic because when I drink too much, I get sick before I can get really bombed.
- Alcoholics look like sloppy drunks; I never look like that, so I can't be addicted.
- I only drink to please my friends; I can stop whenever I want to.
- Alcoholism doesn't run in my family.
- I never drink on school nights.
- I only drink on weekends.
- I only drink at parties.

All these statements may be true, yet you still may have an alcohol problem. If you have any doubts, talk about it with someone you trust.

A TO Z ENTRIES

▉ ADVERTISING AND COUNTERADVERTISING CAMPAIGNS

Attempts to reach a target market by designing a series of advertisements and placing them in various media. As a typical teenager, you have seen many TV commercials promoting beer. You've seen good-looking, healthy young actors on the TV screen who seem to know how to enjoy life—and they are depicted drinking beer. They never feel lonely or awkward. They always are surrounded by happy, supportive friends.

How much do these ads influence you, or other teenagers? Experts disagree. Yet whether or not the ads influence *most* people, *you* can maintain your own independence if you remain critically aware of the "information" you receive about alcohol.

ARE TEENS TARGETED?

For years, critics have accused the makers of beer and other alcoholic beverages of deliberately promoting their products to the underage market. Are they right?

No one has actually proven that the industry is in fact trying to get kids to drink—or to drink more than they already do. Furthermore, there is no clear-cut evidence that the ads actually do influence drinking behavior.

Everyone agrees, however, that the average teenager is exposed to several hundred alcohol commercials every year. The industry-wide advertising budget to promote alcohol drinking was more than $1.2 billion per year in the late 1990s, according to industry figures reported to the Federal Trade Commission. Beer companies alone spent more than $700 million a year on television and radio advertising in 2000, according to the Center for Science in the Public Interest, an advocacy group.

The alcohol industry says that it does not broadcast ads for beer and wine during programs where more than half the viewers are under 21. Yet teens frequently watch programs broadcast after 9 P.M., which are supposedly aimed at adults. They also watch sporting events; during the 1998 Super Bowl, a full 23 minutes of beer ads were shown.

According to an August 2002 report in *Alcoholism & Drug Abuse Weekly*, 77 percent of kids aged 12–18 view television after 9 P.M. Ads in these time slots often are quite entertaining: 73 percent of a sample group of 750 teens remembered seeing alcohol ads, and most of them could even remember the brand names that were advertised.

In December 2002, the Center on Alcohol Marketing and Youth (CAMY) at Georgetown University found that alcohol was advertised on 13 of the 15 shows most popular with the teen demographic, or population-group. In fact, CAMY found that teens between 12 and 20 see more commercials for beer, malt drinks, and other alcoholic beverages than for kid-oriented products such as chewing gum or snacks.

The hidden message

Commercials for distilled spirits, such as whiskey, gin, and vodka, do not appear on American TV, yet commercials for beer and wine do. This creates a mistaken assumption that there is little risk involved in drinking beer or wine. In fact, all these products are alcoholic beverages, and they all have similar effects on the mind and body.

The various pre-mixed beverages that appear on the market every now and then may cause the most confusion. For example, in the 1980s, the alcohol industry began heavily marketing wine coolers via TV commercials.

Coolers are blends of wine and ingredients such as fruit juice that hide the taste of alcohol. They have a lower alcohol *percentage* than wine (6 percent compared with more than 13 percent for most wines). However, the average cooler bottle holds at least twice as much liquid as a wine glass, so the amount of alcohol in one serving is about the same. In other words, coolers are alcoholic beverages in every sense of the word, although many kids don't know that. For example, a 1996 survey of 70,000 kids in grades 4 to 6 conducted by the Texas Commission on Alcohol and Drug Abuse found that coolers were considered the least dangerous type of alcoholic beverage.

Wine coolers represent a far smaller portion of the alcohol market than beer. Beer commercials often use themes and images that kids find especially appealing. Hip, talking frogs and cute racing squirrels are right at home in children's programming but send mixed messages in ads used to promote beer. Some commercials show rugged-looking men and women scaling mountain cliffs or racing bikes over the roughest terrain. These ads may send a "hidden" message that drinking beer makes the viewer strong and tough.

Other commercials use sex appeal. Of course, most teenagers understand that drinking beer does not make boys suddenly attractive to beautiful women. Yet the question is: Do clever ads appeal to one's good sense—or to one's emotions?

The placement of alcohol commercials is an issue too. Kids tend to be fans of sports and music programs, many of which have alcohol sponsors. Advertisers build on kids' loyalty to their favorite stars, and transfer that appeal to the product they are advertising.

A 1994 study in the *American Journal of Public Health* reported an interesting connection between ads and what kids actually thought about drinking. The kids who were most aware of beer advertising were more likely to have favorable notions of drinking, and to express their intention to drink. The authors concluded that "alcohol advertising may pre-dispose young people to drinking."

Not just TV
College campuses have one feature in common with popular TV shows—a mixed age group. While most freshmen, sophomores, and juniors are underage, the typical college also enrolls many graduate students, enough to make up a sizable market for advertisers. This provides an "in" for advertisers and promoters, who are legally entitled to advertise to the over-21 set. Brewers and beer distributors were spending $20 million a year on marketing to colleges in the 1990s, much of it on sponsorship of sporting events. However, by 2001, the majority of colleges told a National Collegiate Athletic Association survey that they no longer accepted alcohol ads at sporting events.

The growth of the Internet has provided another channel for alcohol marketing to reach kids. Brewers and distillers have put up some of the most exciting Web sites, with video, sound effects, interactive games, and product promotions.

WHAT SHOULD GOVERNMENT DO?
The government takes a much lower profile with alcohol advertising than it does with tobacco. One reason is that tobacco is harmful to all users, while alcohol may be used safely by some people.

Now and then, however, public-interest groups have called on the government to get involved. That happened in 1996, after the distilled spirits industry dropped its voluntary ban on TV and radio ads. The industry's Distilled Spirits Council (DISCUS) claimed that current practices discriminated against their companies in favor of beer brewers and wine manufacturers.

Their decision caused a public uproar. Hundreds of public-interest groups appealed to the Federal Communications Commission to intervene, and bills were proposed in Congress. In the end, most broadcasters refused the ads, and the voluntary ban remains in effect.

"COUNTERATTACK"
Given the apparent success of anti-smoking ads, some activists have begun calling for alcohol counteradvertising. They want to show ads

that feature cool kids having fun *without* alcohol. According to a 2002 study by the National Institute on Alcohol Abuse and Alcoholism (NIAAA), "There is an increasing body of literature that suggests that alcohol counteradvertising is effective in reducing the alcohol consumption of teenagers and young adults."

THE ALCOHOL INDUSTRY'S VIEW

The alcohol industry consistently denies that it targets the under-21 age group, claiming that it does not want to waste money appealing to people who cannot legally buy their products. In March 2003, a spokesperson for DISCUS said, "Advertising, whether someone is of age or not, affects what they might choose to drink, not whether they drink."

Some independent observers agree. In 1997 an article appeared in *Priorities*, a reputable journal that sometimes takes controversial stands on public-health issues. The title of the article says it all: "Alcohol Advertising Does Not Promote Underage Drinking." The author claims that public fears that TV ads lead to teen alcohol abuse have not been backed up by research. He prefers to rely on the natural skepticism of young people as a defense against any hidden messages in the ads. He even speculates that advertising bans could backfire, since some kids seem to resent any attempt by grownups to "tell them what to do."

IT'S UP TO YOU

The controversy over alcohol advertising probably will be around for a long time to come, but the bottom line for teens is simple. Go ahead and laugh at the funny commercial—just don't forget all the facts you are learning about the very real risks of underage drinking. When the time comes for you to decide, remember that it is not cool to let anyone else make your decision for you, whether that is a real-life friend or an animated puppet on the TV screen.

See also: Drinking on College Campuses

■ ALCOHOL, HISTORY OF

Throughout recorded history, and probably long before, people have been making and drinking alcoholic beverages. Historians do not know where they were first discovered, but it is easy to guess how it might have happened.

Wild fruits, berries, and honey exposed to the air in warm weather naturally ferment—the sugar turns to alcohol and carbon dioxide. The yeast that helps the process along is floating in the air. For primitive people, food was always scarce. Sooner or later, some cave dwellers would have been willing to try a concoction they discovered in the woods that looked, smelled, and tasted spoiled. Almost every primitive people ever encountered has brewed beer or made wine. In the entire world, only the Polynesians and the Native Americans of the present-day United States and Canada did not discover and use alcohol on their own.

Once people invented writing and the arts, the record became clearer. Every ancient civilization left behind written evidence of alcoholic beverages.

The earliest civilizations in the ancient Near East, from Egypt to Mesopotamia, brewed beer from grains. Enterprising people sold the beverage in taverns, but rulers often distributed it free to citizens during religious festivals. Artists painted brewing scenes on walls and pottery. Archeologists have even found traces (tiny amounts) of beer still clinging to 5,000-year-old clay pitchers.

Ancient Hindu books from almost that far back tell about mead, a wine made from honey. Chinese people under the Shang dynasty more than 3,000 years ago drank beer, and may have drunk grape wine as well. In Mexico and Peru, long before the Spanish conquest, beer was made from corn. In Africa, grains, fruits, honey, and palm sap were used as raw materials for beer and wine.

Winemaking has been around for many thousands of years. But for most of history, beer was the most popular drink; in many countries, including the United States, it still is. The raw materials for beer—mainly grains, such as barley or corn—were much more common than grapes. Also, beer was quicker to make and easier to store.

Until the time of the Greeks, wine was considered an elite product, used in sacrifices to the gods or on ceremonial occasions by kings and their associates. By the time of the Romans, however, farmers were growing grapevines all across the Roman and Persian Empires. When the early Christian Church adopted wine for its central sacrament, wine had become perhaps the most popular alcoholic beverage. However, most people drank wine (naturally 8 to 12 percent alcohol) diluted by 50 percent with water.

Distilled spirits or liquors are a more recent invention. They do not occur naturally and did not become common until the late Middle

Ages—after around A.D. 1200. These beverages, with their much higher alcohol content, caused many social problems and helped change the way many people viewed alcohol.

HISTORICAL USES

As far as historians can tell, people used—and abused—alcohol in the past in some of the same ways as they do today: for relaxation, to bring people together at social and religious events and celebrations, to give people "courage" to face unavoidable tasks, and to drown out sorrows and failures.

Alcohol was also used for medicinal purposes in ancient times, much more so than today. Doctors prescribed it to deaden pain when few other painkillers were known or available. Sumerian and Egyptian doctors wrote down recipes for beer-and-herb mixtures as treatments for various ailments.

Alcoholic beverages may have supplied much-needed nutrition as well. Early beer, less refined than today's, may have contained more starch and other nutrients; besides, beer can be stored easily and preserved for times of scarcity, as during the winter in northern regions. Today's alcoholic beverages, however, are a poor supply of nutrition.

Alcoholic beverages were also widely used as libations, poured offerings to the gods, often including special gods and goddesses of beer and wine. The Bible records that Moses provided for daily libations of wine in the Temple.

Large quantities of wine or beer were also handed out and consumed at religious or civic festivals, where drunkenness and wild dancing was sometimes considered holy. It was a way for people to achieve ecstasy and unite with the spirit world. The notorious bacchanalias, festivals to the wine god Bacchus, eventually became so destructive that the Roman Senate banned them from all of Italy.

Alcohol abuse as known today was also known to the ancient world. Literature from all over the world condemned drunkenness as a cause of immorality and violence; Bible stories about Noah and Lot are good examples. Stories and poetry sometimes depicted people who would today be called alcohol dependent or **alcoholics**, and ancient doctors knew about the health dangers of alcohol abuse.

Nevertheless, alcohol was rarely considered a major problem for society as a whole until the spread of cheap distilled spirits (mostly gin) in Europe in the 1600s and 1700s. Before then, drunkenness had usually been confined to special occasions, or kept hidden in people's homes.

But in the growing cities of the early modern era, with their large, crowded populations, private behavior became everybody's business. Many people accustomed to beer, with its low alcohol content, could not handle the 45-percent alcohol content of gin and other distilled spirits.

As a result of the perceived harm to families and communities, a **temperance movement** began to emerge in England in the 18th century, centered on the independent churches. The movement advocated a "temperate" or moderate use of alcohol.

In England's American colonies, rum from the West Indies was popular, along with gin and whiskey. As in England, many American civic and church leaders began to preach against the abuse of alcohol—or even against its use in any amount. This was the start of what became the **prohibition** movement, an organized ban on the drinking of any alcohol.

LAWS CONTROLLING ALCOHOL USE AND PROHIBITION

Public laws and regulations to control the use and abuse of alcohol are almost as old as the beverages themselves. The famous Hammurabi Code, a series of laws issued by the Babylonian King Hammurabi around 1800 B.C., included measures such as fixing prices and controlling the sale of alcohol by taverns. In ancient Egypt, priests preached against overdrinking.

When the drinking of alcohol outside of religious occasions began to spread in ancient China, the government tried to impose prohibition, but it was never successfully enforced. Various rulers of ancient Persia, Greece, and Rome also tried to control or limit alcohol abuse.

Some of the major world religions have banned alcohol among their followers, though they have not always succeeded in enforcing the ban. For example, Buddhism has advised against alcohol since its start 2,500 years ago, yet alcohol is still widely used among the Buddhist peoples of south and east Asia. In India, the Hindu faith teaches that alcohol is impure. But despite the appeals for prohibition by Mahatma Gandhi and other leaders, only members of the elite Brahmin caste generally abstain from alcohol.

The Koran, the sacred text of the Muslim religion, strictly bans all alcohol. That ban has probably been the most successful prohibition effort in history. Alcohol is not easy to find in some Arab countries to this day. Even so, drinking is not unknown in most Muslim countries and is widespread in some.

In the modern world, nearly every country has laws to control the production, sale, and consumption of alcohol, to ensure a source of steady tax income for the government as well as to control and limit abuses. These practices began in England in the mid-1700s, when the government passed many laws to restrict the times and places that gin could be sold. The laws raised taxes on gin and tried to dilute its alcohol content. These measures were largely successful; England went back to its beer- and ale-drinking traditions, which it preserves to the present day.

The most famous attempt to limit drinking was the Eighteenth, or Prohibition, Amendment to the U.S. Constitution, passed in 1919. That "great experiment" is discussed in the entry on "Law and Drinking."

PRODUCTION OF ALCOHOL

Manufacturers all over the world offer a huge, confusing variety of alcoholic beverages for sale. Despite all those labels, all the products fall into only three basic categories: wine, beer, and liquor, or distilled spirits.

Wine

Wine (typically around 12 or 13 percent alcohol) is usually made from grapes, but other fruits can be used as well. (Apple cider is, strictly speaking, a kind of wine.) Winemakers use thousands of different grape varieties, which all derive from the same species of grape. Most

---

DID YOU KNOW?

One Drink Equals . . .

12 ounces of beer (12-ounce bottle or can)

12 ounces of wine cooler (standard bottle)

5 ounces of wine (standard wine glass)

3 ounces of sherry or port (small wine glass)

1.5 ounces of brandy (standard shot glass)

1.5 ounces of 80-proof liquor (standard shot glass)

1 ounce of 120-proof liquor (two-thirds standard shot glass)

1.5–3 ounces of liqueur (check the label!)

Source: Indiana Prevention Resource Center, 2004.

of the grape's juice is naturally white: The color in red and rose wines comes primarily from the skin.

Grapes are harvested, crushed, and poured into vats or barrels, where natural **fermentation,** a natural process in which sugar chemically turns into alcohol, takes place due to yeast in the grapes; extra sugar and yeast are sometimes added. During fermentation, much of the sugar turns to alcohol and carbon dioxide, which is usually allowed to evaporate.

Alcohol is toxic to yeast, so fermentation is a self-limiting process: It stops as soon as the alcohol reaches a concentration of 10 to 15 percent, which can happen over a few days or up to several weeks, depending on the type of wine. Sparkling wines, such as champagne, go through a second fermentation in the bottle, with sugar and yeast added to produce more carbon dioxide. Fortified wines, such as sherry and port, have brandy added to them to increase the percentage of alcohol, to as much as 23 percent. Liqueurs, or aperitifs, are sweet heavy wines to which herbs and other ingredients, such as quinine, are added for flavor. Wine coolers are carbonated blends of white wine and citrus juices.

Not long ago, France was the largest producer of wine in the world, followed by Italy, with French wines regarded as the best. But with the growth of globalization and the spread of technology, many other countries and regions have become major producers and exporters of wine, including California in the United States, several South American and eastern European countries, South Africa, and Australia.

Fact Or Fiction?

In France, where drinking wine with meals is an honored part of the culture, there is no alcoholism.

Fact: Research proves this statement false. There are about two million alcoholics in France, according to recent research, roughly the same percentage of the population as in the United States. With so many people abusing alcohol, France suffers many of the alcohol-related problems Americans do: More than one third of all motor vehicle crash deaths, a quarter of suicides, and about one half of all homicides involve the beverage. It is interesting to note that French people have been drinking less wine in recent years, maybe because of campaigns aimed at kids with the message, "How do you look when you're drunk?"

Beer

Beer (ranging from 4 to more than 6 percent alcohol) can be made from any cereal grain, most often barley but also wheat, rice, or corn, or from starchy roots such as sweet potatoes. Unlike the sugar in grapes, the starch in grain does not ferment on its own. It needs to be turned into sugar by a process called malting.

For malting, the grain is first allowed to germinate in water (the seeds begin to grow into tiny plants). The germinated grain, or *malt*, is then cracked (separated from the husk), dried, and mashed into hot water, where it turns into sugar.

Brewers then add hops, an aromatic plant, for flavor, color, and aroma. Finally, they add yeast to promote fermentation of the sugar into alcohol. Fermentation can take up to several months.

Brewers produce various types of beer and ale (a category of beer) using different techniques. They can use different grains as raw material; add a variety of unmalted grains and vary the water temperature during the mashing step; use different types of yeast during fermentation to control carbonation; add various flavoring ingredients just before bottling; and allow the product to age more or less in the bottle before refrigeration or sale. Draft beer is beer that is not pasteurized (heated to kill germs); it must be kept refrigerated throughout the distribution path, unlike pasteurized beer, which can be stored safely at room temperature.

Q & A

Question: Is there any alcohol in "nonalcoholic" beer, and is there any risk involved in drinking this product?

Answer: Nonalcoholic beers are made from alcoholic beer. The alcohol is removed through evaporation, but a small amount does remain in the product—up to one-half of 1 percent. For people without a history of alcohol abuse, there should not be any problem drinking a cold, tasty "near beer." However, for alcoholics, the smell of nonalcoholic beer may trigger cravings for the real beverage. A study reported in the November 1999 issue of *Alcoholism: Clinical and*

Experimental Research found that olfactory cues (smells) can easily trigger cravings for alcohol.

Liquor

Liquors, or distilled spirits (with widely ranging alcohol content of up to 90 percent), are all produced by the same two-step technique. The process was discovered more than 2,000 years ago but did not become widely adopted until around the year A.D. 1600.

The first step is fermentation, usually with grains as the initial raw material. The second step is distillation, a process during which the distiller boils the fermented mash. The boiling yields a steam of alcohol and flavorings; the steam rises into another, cooler container, where it condenses back into liquor. Since much of the nonalcoholic liquid stays behind, the liquor has a much higher alcohol content.

Whiskeys are various grain liquors traditionally aged for a period of years in oak barrels. Slight differences in processing, and different alcohol percentages, account for the different tastes and textures. Bourbon is made largely from corn and aged in barrels that have been charred. Scotch is usually exposed to peat smoke. Rye is produced largely from rye grain, and corn liquor is produced mostly from corn.

Vodka, made from potatoes or grain, generally has the same alcohol content as whiskey (roughly 40–50 percent), but it is filtered through charcoal to remove color and taste. Gin is flavored with juniper berries. Brandy and cognac are distilled from grape wine. Rum is made from sugarcane or molasses, and tequila from the agave plant.

Every country and people in the world has its own variations of liquors, with different additives, mixers, and raw materials. The alcohol concentration can vary greatly, but is always much greater than that in beer or wine. In the United States, alcohol is labeled with its **proof**, which is twice its alcohol percentage by volume. In other words, liquor labeled as 80-proof is 40 percent alcohol by volume. Remember, that is more than *three times* as potent as most wines and *seven times* as potent as beer.

See also: Effects on the Body; Law and Drinking, The

FURTHER READING
Harriet Lembeck. *Grossman's Cyclopedia: The Concise Guide to Wines, Beers, and Spirits.* Philadelphia, PA: Running Press, 2002.

Roderick Phillips. *A Short History of Wine.* New York: Ecco, 2000.
Gregg Smith. *Beer: A History of Suds and Civilization from Mesopotamia to Microbreweries.* New York: Avon, 1995.

■ ALCOHOL ABUSE, THE RISKS OF

Alcohol abuse refers to the potential "down side" or consequences of a drinking pattern that leads to **intoxication** or **addiction** causing one or more behavior problems. You have probably heard the expression "calculated risk." Most of the choices people make in life involve a price they have to pay if things go wrong. As teenagers leave childhood behind and begin to think and act like adults, they may find it useful to calculate, or think through, the benefits and risks of possible behaviors. Alcohol abuse is one of those behaviors.

The problem behaviors that can result from alcohol abuse can include failure to live up to your responsibilities; drinking under dangerous conditions; getting in frequent trouble with the law; and having alcohol-related problems with a spouse or friend.

Of course, people do not stop a hundred times a day to do the calculations. At any point in their lives, most people do what is routine. For example, adults who have mastered the art of drinking in moderation do not need to stop and think each time they have a glass of wine with dinner. Other adults, who have decided to abstain from any alcohol, do not bother to rethink the issue every time someone offers them a drink. And, unfortunately, **alcoholics** may feel powerless to change their unhealthy behavior patterns. Young people, however, who have not yet settled into regular behavior patterns, can learn about the risks and do their own calculations. They should be aware that the decisions they make can eventually become habits.

THE RISK OF INJURY

According to the Centers for Disease Control and Prevention (CDC), more than 150,000 Americans die every year from trauma to the body—in other words, injury. Trauma is the leading cause of death for people aged one to 44. Millions more suffer nonfatal injuries—one out of three individuals, according to the CDC. Sometimes it seems as if the world is one big booby trap, ready to go off without warning.

In almost every case, physicians or emergency staff can find an immediate cause for these deaths: for example, a vehicle crash, fire, poisoning, or deliberate act of violence. But too often, the real under-lying cause is alcohol use or alcohol abuse, meaning a pattern of drinking that results in at least one of these behaviors: failure to ful-fill major responsibilities; drinking in dangerous situations, for exam-ple, when driving; having alcohol-related legal problems; having alcohol-related relationship problems.

In June 1999, the *Annals of Emergency Medicine* published a study conducted at the Johns Hopkins School of Public Health, which found that "alcohol is often an important factor" in fatal injuries of all kinds. Compiling multiyear data from medical examiners around the country, the study found that 31.5 percent of homicide victims were intoxicated at the time of death, with a BAL, or **blood alcohol level** (percentage of alcohol in the bloodstream), of at least .10. Similarly, the victims of 31 percent of unintentional injury deaths (deaths caused by negligent or careless actions) and 22 percent of suicide deaths were intoxicated at the time of death.

The problem is a longstanding one. According to a 1989 "Alcohol Alert" from the National Institute of Alcohol Abuse and Alcoholism, surveys also showed a high percentage of injuries involving people with high BALs. Intoxicated individuals caused some 40–50 percent of motor vehicle fatalities (deaths), 25–35 percent of nonfatal motor vehicle injuries, 64 percent of fires and burns, 48 percent of frostbite and hypothermia (very low body temperature, generally resulting from passing out or sleeping outdoors in cold weather), and 20 per-cent of suicides.

Furthermore, most studies show that the alcohol-related injuries tend to be the more serious ones. The reasons are clear. Alcohol, even at moderate levels, can weaken people's judgment, slow down their reaction times, and make them clumsy and uncoordinated. That is why no supervisor with any sense allows a worker to operate dan-gerous machinery while under the influence of alcohol.

Q & A

Question: We know that people who operate machinery in the workplace should not drink. What about operating machinery for recreation? For example, what about boating?

Answer: More than half of all recreational boating deaths involve alcohol. According to the U.S. Coast Guard, "a boat operator with a blood alcohol concentration above .10 is ten times more likely to be killed in a boating accident than a boater with a zero blood alcohol concentration." A little bit of alcohol may actually be more dangerous for boaters than for automobile drivers. Sun, wind, noise, vibration, and boat motion can enhance the effects of alcohol. You should be alert when operating *any* vehicle.

RISKS IN THE EMERGENCY ROOM

Being sober is no guarantee that you will always avoid injury. Also, people who have been drinking might become trauma victims through events beyond their control. But even if alcohol did not cause an injury, drinking entails an additional risk for those who are injured: It can get in the way of a doctor making a quick, accurate diagnosis.

When a trauma victim turns up at a hospital emergency room (ER) with a bruise on the forehead, slurred speech, and an unsteady gait, the medical staff would normally suspect a serious head injury. But when they get a strong whiff of alcohol as they approach the victim, they suddenly see a different picture. They should still check for serious injury, but in the real, high-pressure world of an ER, some staff might be tempted to lead the victim to a bed to "sleep it off" while they deal with other emergencies.

If a patient who has been drinking does *not* show signs of intoxication in the ER, that can be dangerous too. Alcohol does not mix well with many standard medications, including antibiotics and painkillers. If the patient is unconscious, confused, or fails to tell staff that he or she has been drinking, the wrong drug may be administered, with dangerous results.

THE RISK OF UNINTENDED DEATH

Some unlucky people are deathly allergic to even one peanut. Everyone else, fortunately, can eat as many as they could possibly want and still suffer no more than a bellyache. The reverse is true of alcohol. Almost no one is truly allergic to the substance, but *anyone* can get seriously ill or even die if he or she drinks too fast, too much, or in combination with certain other substances.

Binge drinking

Regular heavy drinking can be dangerous to your health. Binge drinking, when someone has five or more drinks on one occasion, is an injury waiting to happen. But chugging, drinking a large quantity in a short period of time, can kill.

As a general rule, the liver of an average person can metabolize, or break down, the alcohol in one drink in about an hour. People who drink more than one drink an hour, whether shots of whiskey or bottles of beer, are overloading their bloodstreams with alcohol. The more they put into their systems, the higher their blood alcohol level.

When your BAL goes above .08 (which may happen after just a few standard-sized drinks), you are considered unfit to drive in most states (although some people may be unfit to drive at lower levels too). As the level rises (and it surely does if you drink too fast), the toxic (poisonous) effects of alcohol on the brain and nervous system start to kick in. When your BAL hits .25, you lose your coordination, and you can easily choke on your own vomit if you are alone or if your drinking companions are also intoxicated and unable to help.

When you continue chugging, your BAL can rise above .30, when you could pass out. At .35, your breathing may stop; without immediate medical care to restore your breathing, you may die. At .40, even if your breathing can be restored, you may suffer permanent brain damage and slip into a coma.

You might think that once you pass out and can no longer continue drinking, you can never reach the deadly levels. Unfortunately, the BAL can keep rising even *after* you stop drinking, as the alcohol in your stomach continues to be absorbed into the bloodstream faster than your body can break it down. If your friends pour coffee into you, push you into a cold shower, or walk you around the room, you might feel a bit more alert, but none of those measures reduces the BAL and the damage it can cause. If someone you know passes out after chugging, you should seek immediate medical attention.

Fact Or Fiction?

"If my friend has had so much to drink he's passed out, he can be revived if I make him drink lots of coffee."

Fact: Wrong. Coffee may help keep your friend awake, but it will have no impact on his blood alcohol level. If he has had so much alcohol to drink that he passes out, he may be in danger. If you are reasonably sober, keep a very close watch to make sure he continues to breathe normally, and make sure he's lying on his side or upright to keep him from choking on his own vomit. If you are not in a condition to monitor your friend, you should get help from someone who can.

Chugging

Chugging means drinking a large amount of alcohol in as short a time as possible. It is relatively rare among adults, but all too common among the underage. Underage drinkers are more likely to engage in the activity for several reasons, apart from lack of experience and lack of knowledge. Teenagers know they are not allowed to buy alcohol when attending a party, concert, or sporting event. To compensate, some kids chug down several drinks before they arrive at their destination, as if their stomachs were fuel tanks that they can tap as needed in the course of an evening.

But it doesn't work that way at all. Instead, *all* the alcohol is absorbed into the blood in a matter of an hour or so. Instead of a steady high, these young drinkers can expect a brief roller-coaster ride, with extreme intoxication followed by physical or mental collapse.

Kids who feel insecure may try to impress friends with their ability to hold their liquor. And kids who want to be accepted by a club or fraternity—or by any crowd of other kids—may calculate that the goal is worth accepting the challenge to chug. If they understood that the risk is brain damage or death, would the calculation come out the same?

Even modest amounts of alcohol can kill when combined with certain prescription or over-the-counter medications or with illicit drugs. At the very least, if you are fighting a bacterial infection, alcohol can make antibiotics lose their effect in your system, leading to a surge in the bacteria you are trying to fight. At the worst, alcohol can intensify the effects of certain other drugs, causing unpredictable damage to vital body systems.

When mixing drugs and alcohol, a little bit of knowledge can be a dangerous thing. A friend may tell you that mixing alcohol with a particular drug gives you a stronger high and can't harm you. Perhaps your friend has done it once or twice and lived to tell the tale. But remember, before any drug can be legally sold, it is tested on thousands of people for a period of several years, and every bad reaction is carefully recorded. Unless your friend's concoction has undergone such scrutiny, it cannot be trusted. Play it safe and avoid taking unnecessary risks.

DOMESTIC ABUSE

Domestic abuse, the regular mistreatment of one family member or romantic partner by another, is one of the more heartbreaking phenomena often associated with problem drinking. A study in the December 1999 *New England Journal of Medicine* reported that alcohol abuse was the greatest single risk factor causing injuries to female victims of domestic violence. But the problem goes well beyond the headline-grabbing crimes of violence. Abuse can include frightening verbal assaults, insults and unfair criticism, denial of affection, broken promises, poor supervision, lack of support, or neglect.

Child abuse is a growing problem. The National Clearinghouse on Child Abuse and Neglect Information (NCCANI) of the U.S. Department of Health and Human Services reported that in 2001, more than 900,000 children were "victims of child maltreatment"—a rate of 12.4 out of every 1,000 kids. Of these, 57 percent suffered neglect, 19 percent physical abuse, 10 percent sexual abuse, and 7 percent psychological maltreatment.

In 1999, the National Center on Addiction and Substance Abuse (CASA) at Columbia University stated that alcohol and drug abuse among parents are the most important causes of the rise in child abuse and neglect in recent years. The center found that parents who abuse drugs or alcohol are 2.7 times more likely to abuse their kids, and more than 4 times more likely to neglect them. The NCCANI reported in 2003 that an earlier (1989) study found that alcohol and drug abuse by parents were involved in some 70 percent of child neglect cases in many urban areas.

Substance abuse is not generally the *only* cause of these problems. Other personal or social factors are often involved too, but alcohol makes the problems worse and harder to resolve. A parent whose time and money are devoted to heavy drinking is less likely to carry out his or her responsibilities to spouse and children.

Parental neglect and alcohol abuse are related in another way. Even the best of parents may not be able to protect their children in every situation. However, parents who abuse alcohol are less able to provide their teenage kids with supervision or attention, and poor parental supervision is an important cause of teenage alcohol abuse.

NOT AN EQUAL-OPPORTUNITY DRUG: WOMEN AND ALCOHOL ABUSE

In the past, researchers found that, for Americans as a whole, men are twice as likely as women to suffer from alcohol abuse or alcohol dependency. This gap may be disappearing, if behavior among teenagers is any guide. A CASA study in 2002 found that "male and female ninth graders are just as likely to drink (40 percent vs. 41 percent) and to binge drink (22 percent vs. 20 percent)."

Some researchers say that gender equality is in part responsible for this change. Many girls now believe that they do not have to follow old-fashioned ideas about "feminine" behavior. Some may think, "If boys can do it, even though it's illegal and risky, why can't we girls?" Unfortunately, nature is not always fair. Behaviors that are harmful for one gender may be even more harmful for the other. Alcohol abuse is one of those, and the female gender suffers the most.

If a boy and a girl drink the same quantity of alcohol, the girl's BAL is higher, for at least three reasons. To begin with, girls tend to be smaller than boys, at any age group, and body size influences how much alcohol can be safely imbibed. Secondly, boys have more active stomach enzymes, protein chemicals in the stomach that speed up chemical reactions, such as breaking down alcohol before it can be absorbed into the bloodstream. Finally, according to the National Institute on Alcohol Abuse and Alcoholism, even when a man and a woman have the same body size, the man has higher body water content, which dilutes the alcohol to some degree.

The higher BAL has two dangerous consequences: the girl becomes intoxicated sooner than the boy, and her health is more likely to suffer. On the average, American women live several years longer than men. But women alcohol abusers do not benefit from the same advantage—they have higher death rates than male alcohol abusers for several different alcohol-related problems, including liver disease, unintentional injuries, and suicide.

In addition, too much alcohol can upset the delicate balance of hormones that control a woman's reproductive system. This can cause menstrual periods to be irregular or painful, or even to stop altogether. Among pregnant women, it can cause miscarriage. Among older women, it can cause premature menopause.

Heavy drinkers, or people who have five or more drinks per occasion at least five different times a month, often lose calcium, a vital nutrient for bones and all body cells. Alcohol seems to upset the chemical systems that distribute the mineral through the body. Calcium actually drains away from bone tissue and is expelled in urine. This happens with men as well as women, but the consequences seem to be worse for females. Because women have a greater natural risk of osteoporosis, a disease of the bones that can lead to weakness and fractures, the additional damage caused by alcohol can make the difference between a manageable condition and crippling pain.

Some of the social consequences of alcohol abuse—whether by men *or* by women—fall more heavily on women too. Such consequences may include spousal abuse, rape, and unplanned or unprotected sex, which in turn can cause unwanted pregnancy and sexually transmitted diseases.

Alcohol in large, persistent quantities can be devastating to women. On the other hand, *small* amounts of alcohol (one or two drinks a day) may help older women produce estrogen, the basic female hormone, according to a study reported by the National Institute on Alcohol Abuse and Alcoholism in 2001. As a result, moderate women drinkers have a *lower* risk than nondrinkers for osteoporosis and heart disease.

TEENS SPEAK

Girls Are Different, Sometimes

"The worst part is, I finally find a boy I really like, and then we have to break up," Carolynn says. "My parents never tell me what to do, but this time they got scared. And the truth is, I had to agree they're right."

Carolynn had just started her junior year. She was feeling very mature and self-confident after volunteering at a camp for disabled kids, and she was starting to hang out with a nice ("really cute") guy.

The only problem was that Matthew and his friends like to drink. "Every Friday night they get together at Matthew's brother's apartment and work their way through all these six-packs. I told him, 'Sure I drink beer.' But all I ever have is one glass, at my father's barbecues."

That Friday night Carolynn and another girl started in with the guys. "After the second beer I was really buzzed," she remembers. "I was the only one; everyone thought it was funny." She thinks the other girl stopped after two, but

Carolynn wanted to keep up with Matthew—"I can do any-thing a boy can," she remembers thinking.

What she didn't know is that alcohol works faster on women, and it works faster on smaller people. Carolynn is five foot four and weighs 115 pounds; Matthew is a hefty five ten and a half. When you take weight and sex into account, she really had two drinks for every one of his.

"I wound up vomiting in Matthew's lap just before I conked out," she says. She was incoherent when Matthew handed her over to her parents; her mother insisted on tak-ing a picture so she could see herself the next morning. "It's a picture I'll never forget," she promises.

DID YOU KNOW?

The Costs of Alcohol Abuse in the United States, 1998

Category	$ billion	total, $ billion
Medical costs		18.9
Alcohol and drug abuse services	5.5	
Lost earnings		134.2
Premature death	36.5	
Impaired productivity	87.6	
Lost productivity of people in prison	9.1	
Crime victims	1	
Other impacts		31.5
Specialty alcohol services	7.5	
Crime costs (other than productivity)	6.3	
Motor vehicle crashes (other than medical)	5.7	
Fire destruction	1.5	
Grand total		184.6

Source: *The Economic Costs of Alcohol and Drug Abuse in the United States*, U.S. Department of Health and Human Services, National Institute on Alcohol Abuse and Alcoholism, December 2000.

THE SOCIAL COSTS

Economists have tried to calculate the economic cost to society of alcohol abuse. Unfortunately, hospitals and insurance companies do not always keep separate tabulations of illnesses and injuries that are caused, or partly caused, by alcohol abuse; thus, the calculations are really estimates, or educated guesses.

Also, it is impossible to measure how much more productive alcohol abusers could be if they overcame their drinking problems. Nevertheless, in 2000, the U.S. Department of Health and Human Services felt sure enough about the facts to estimate that the cost of alcohol abuse to the U.S. economy in 1998 was $185 billion. The largest component was lost earnings and production in the workplace, figured at $134 billion. Medical costs came to nearly $19 billion, not including $7.5 billion for treatment programs. Alcohol-related crime cost $6.3 billion, while alcohol-related motor vehicle crashes cost $5.7 billion.

How do these costs add up? For starters, alcohol abusers cost employers four times the average amount in sickness and injury benefits. They also have double the normal rate of absence from work—9 percent of heavy drinkers miss work due to hangovers, according to the National Council on Alcohol and Drug Dependency, while 6 percent actually go to work drunk. There is no way to calculate the effects of intoxicated employees on coworker morale and client relations.

If these figures are correct, the annual cost to society is approximately $14,000 for each problem drinker (based on a total of 13 million, according to the 2001 National Household Survey on Drug Abuse). That's an expensive habit.

THE HEALTH COSTS

In 1996, according to the National Institute on Alcohol Abuse and Alcoholism, more than 110,000 people died in the United States from alcohol-related causes, which works out to 32.2 deaths for every 100,000 Americans. This actually shows a substantial improvement over 1979, when the rate was 42.2.

The agency broke down the total into the following leading causes: motor vehicle injuries, 19 percent; murders, 9 percent; suicides, 8 percent; cirrhosis of the liver, 7 percent; and cancer of the esophagus, 7 percent. The other 50 percent represent the large variety of diseases and injuries caused or worsened by alcohol abuse.

WEIGH YOUR RISKS

The short-term benefits of alcohol may be obvious to teenagers experimenting with alcoholic beverages. Alcohol can help people relax and
have a good time, and may make kids feel accepted and part of the
group. The risks, however, are often not immediately apparent. Smart,
mature teenagers will try to weigh the present and future factors
together when making their decisions about this important part of life.

See also: Alcohol and Disease; Alcohol and Violence; Children of
Alcoholics; Drinking and Drugs; Effects on the Body; Sexual Behavior
and Alcohol

FURTHER READING

Cynthia Kuhn, Scott Swartzwelder, Wilkie Wilson. *Just Say Know:
Talking with Kids about Drugs and Alcohol.* New York: Norton, 2002.
Michael T. Windle. *Alcohol Use among Adolescents.* Thousand Oaks,
CA: Sage Publications, 1999.

■ ALCOHOL AND DISEASE

A disease is any impairment or injury to the normal function of an
organism. Alcohol is such a potent substance that few organ or body
systems are immune from its effects. Some of the effects described
above are healthy, but most are not, especially those caused by heavy
or abusive drinking. No doubt you have discovered in school, at
home, and among your friends that when it comes to making decisions, facing challenges, and learning about new things, no situation,
problem, or issue is ever all black or all white, all bad or all good. The
same holds true for alcohol and your health.

There is good news and bad news about alcohol's effects on the
body—especially on the heart, circulatory system (blood), and brain.
First, the good news.

RECENT RESEARCH ON ALCOHOL AND ADULTS

In recent years, some scientists who study alcohol's effects on people's health have gathered evidence that suggests that moderate
drinking for adults—about two to three drinks a day for men, one to
two drinks for women—appears to reduce the risk of heart attacks and
strokes. Moderate drinking appears to raise "good" cholesterol levels,

inhibit blood clotting, increase blood flow, and reduce blood pressure—all factors that contribute to healthy hearts and brains. It may also decrease a person's chances of developing brain-related diseases such as Alzheimer's and Parkinson's.

It's not what's drunk, but when and how

Scientists first believed that drinking red wine in moderation, just a few times a week, was the most likely way to reap beneficial health effects. They based their theory, in part, on the fact that people in heavy wine-drinking countries, such as France, appeared to have fewer heart-related health problems than other populations, despite a diet high in animal fat.

In September 2003 a group of scientists reported in the journal *Nature* that red wine may have some particularly beneficial effects after all. They reported that **resveratrol**, a chemical found abundantly in red wine, had the effect of stimulating long life in yeast plants and might possibly be involved in preventing diseases of aging in humans as well.

In January 2003, the "drinking-in-moderation" theory was expanded dramatically when the results of Harvard's 12-year Health Professional's Follow-Up Study were published. Scientists analyzed the drinking habits and health histories of more than 37,000 male health professionals (doctors, dentists, optometrists, osteopaths, and veterinarians) for more than a decade.

They concluded that individuals who had one to two drinks at least three days a week lowered their risk of heart attack by 32 to 37 percent. Those who drank at that level on at least five days a week had the lowest risk. In contrast, those who drank once or twice a week lowered their risk of heart attack by only 16 percent, and people who didn't drink at all had an *increased* risk of heart attack.

In other words, these experts reported that drinking frequently, but in moderation, may be part of a healthy lifestyle. Does this mean everyone should start consuming up to 14 drinks a week? Not at all. These experts caution that people who do not now drink should not necessarily begin, given all the other impacts of drinking, in particular the risks for people who have never drunk or have stopped drinking in the past.

Studies about alcohol benefits may be biased

Researchers who study the benefits of alcohol focus almost exclusively on older, educated, professional white males who may naturally be inclined to take good care of themselves and who have better access to health education and preventive healthcare. In research terms, this is called a *built-in bias*. These characteristics make these people a select population group that cannot be fairly compared to other groups, especially young people and women.

When it comes to teenagers, for example, the brain—particularly the portions of the brain responsible for learning, memory, and decision making—continues to develop through young adulthood. And this younger "learning" brain is very sensitive to the damaging effects of alcohol.

Scientists have demonstrated in problem-solving situations that consuming the equivalent of just one drink can impair learning ability in young drinkers up to the age of 25. The same amount of alcohol may show no effect on older people's brains in similar situations. In other words, you and your brain (and for that matter, the rest of your body) may have a lot of growing to do before you can think about making "healthy drinking" a part of your life!

Moderate drinking is a relative term

Despite the evidence that moderate daily drinking may be good for one's health, this theory does not hold up for developing adolescents, teens, and young adults, whose brains and other organs are especially vulnerable to the effects of alcohol.

The phrase *moderate drinking* is a very relative term: That is to say, every individual reacts to alcohol uniquely. What's "moderate" for your parents or a friend may be excessive and damaging for you. In fact, many people who develop serious liver damage from drinking too much tell their doctors that they are only moderate drinkers and deny ever having been drunk.

Fact Or Fiction?

Men and women are not equal when it comes to drinking.

Fact: This is true. Men who consume two to three drinks a day may reduce their risk for heart attack and stroke by as much as 37 percent. Yet women who consume two or more drinks a day may increase their risk of breast cancer by as much as 41 percent. Women drinkers also develop alcohol-related brain, heart, and liver damage much faster than comparable male drinkers, even when drinking less alcohol than men.

People who say alcohol "goes right to your head" (meaning, your brain) are right. At least, that's where you first feel the effects of alcohol. But alcohol also goes to every other organ and cell in your body. It uses your bloodstream to make the trip.

THE BLOODSTREAM: ALCOHOL'S SUPERHIGHWAY

Your body digests, or slowly breaks down, most of the food you eat into nutrients, which are absorbed by the body, and waste materials, which are eliminated.

Unlike food, alcohol is *not* digested. When you drink, alcohol passes directly into your bloodstream through the cells of your digestive tract. It begins its journey in your mouth and throat (where 5 percent of the alcohol in a drink enters the bloodstream within seconds), travels on to your stomach (where 25 percent is absorbed within minutes), and ends in your small intestine (where 70 percent is absorbed within an hour).

It takes from 30 minutes (on an empty stomach) to 60 minutes (on a full stomach) for all the alcohol in one drink to enter your bloodstream. Once alcohol is there, the heart circulates it, via your blood, to all parts of your body. The greatest amounts of alcohol go to those organs that receive the biggest supplies of blood—your brain, liver, and kidneys.

The largest of these organs, the liver, has the vital task of metabolizing, or breaking down, alcohol and removing it from your bloodstream quickly and efficiently. The liver can do this at the rate of about one drink an hour. If you consume more than one drink in an hour, the liver becomes overworked and cannot metabolize all the alcohol in your body.

The more you drink, and the more quickly you drink, the less efficiently your liver works. The result is that larger quantities·of alcohol remain in your bloodstream for a longer time. Because alcohol travels to and affects all parts of your body, this type of drinking—too much, too quickly—can cause severe health problems for your body.

Occasional episodes of this type of drinking can cause minor, short-term health problems; but even one episode of **chugging**, or drinking one drink after another, can put you in the hospital. A regular pattern of overdrinking can have serious, long-term health consequences. Take a brief look at some of these potential short- and long-term health problems, starting with the gastrointestinal (GI) tract.

ALCOHOL AND YOUR GI TRACT

Alcohol irritates the lining of your mouth, throat, esophagus (the "tube" in which food travels), stomach, and intestines. Possible short-term or minor health problems include nausea, vomiting, diarrhea, heartburn (also known as GERD. or gastroesophageal reflux disease), gastritis (inflammation of the stomach lining), ulcers, and irritable bowel syndrome (IBS).

Frequent alcohol use damages the delicate linings of the GI tract and increases the risk of mouth and esophageal cancers, especially if you smoke. In fact, alcohol has been labeled a "co-carcinogen" because it works together with tobacco to significantly increase the risk of certain cancers. For example, Harvard Medical School's Consumer Health Information Service reported in 2001 that more than 80 percent of mouth and esophageal cancers are the result of alcohol and tobacco use. Frequent alcohol use also may increase the risk of stomach, colon, and rectal cancers.

Your pancreas, the organ that produces insulin and helps your body digest food and process sugar, is very sensitive to alcohol's effects. Pancreatitis, an inflamed and painful pancreas, is one of the most common results of frequent alcohol use.

ALCOHOL, YOUR LIVER, AND CIRRHOSIS

The liver breaks down alcohol and removes it from your bloodstream at a relatively slow rate (one drink in one hour). Consequently, overloading the liver with too much alcohol on a regular basis has serious effects on how well that organ functions. Because the liver acts as the body's primary filter for other toxins, drugs, and substances, a liver badly damaged by alcohol affects every system in your body. Once the liver stops functioning, the body quickly dies.

Scientists still do not know exactly *how* alcohol damages the liver, but they know it does, and they know the damage occurs during the breaking-down process. Early signs of alcohol-related liver damage include alcoholic hepatitis, an inflammation of liver tissue that can cause nausea, vomiting, and fatigue. A fatty liver is another early sign of liver damage. Normally, the liver breaks down fat to produce energy for the body, but if the liver is overtaxed with breaking down alcohol, it burns the alcohol as energy instead and allows fat to build up in the liver.

Mild liver damage can be reversed—if you stop drinking—because the liver has the remarkable ability to regenerate itself. However, if frequent drinking continues, the overworked liver develops a network of scar tissue. This is called cirrhosis of the liver, and it is irreversible. Unless you have a liver transplant, cirrhosis leads to complete liver failure and premature death.

Q & A

Question: Is it possible to drown in your own vomit?

Answer: Usually, when you drink too much too quickly, a valve in your stomach begins to contract rapidly and you vomit—often more than once! This is your body's way of protecting itself from alcohol's **toxic** (poisonous) effects. If you really overdo it, however, this protective mechanism may stop working properly. If you then pass out or fall asleep and your body later tries to eliminate the alcohol as vomit, the vomit may back up into your lungs and "drown" you. Although this does not happen frequently, it is not rare. The medical term for the condition is diffuse pulmonary edema.

ALCOHOL, YOUR HEART, AND YOUR BLOOD

Frequent alcohol use raises blood pressure and heart rate, both of which make the heart work much harder to pump blood through the body. Higher blood pressure can cause a variety of problems and often needs to be controlled with medication.

Another, less common effect of frequent alcohol use is a condition called alcoholic cardiomyopathy, or "beer drinker's heart." In this disease, caused by years of excessive alcohol consumption, the heart muscle is inflamed and weakened. In advanced cases, the heart can no longer pump blood.

The major components of blood are red blood cells and white blood cells. They, too, are vulnerable to the damaging effects of alcohol. Red blood cells carry oxygen and hemoglobin, which contains iron, to all parts of the body and remove waste materials during circulation. When red blood cells are damaged by alcohol, they become sticky and cling together. This slows the blood's circulation, deprives organs and tissues of vital oxygen, and encourages blood clotting.

White blood cells are the great infection fighters and the key defensive players in your body's immune system. Some white blood cells produce antibodies that destroy infecting bacteria and viruses; others attack and kill infections directly (these are called "killer white cells"). White blood cells, which have a short life, are constantly reproducing themselves to fight infection. Alcohol damages white blood cells in three ways: it reduces the ability of the cells to create antibodies to fight infections, it impairs the process of blood cell reproduction, and it slows down the infection-fighting action of killer white cells. Damaged white blood cells make for a weak immune system.

Alcohol also damages the immune system by keeping the body from absorbing enough vitamins, minerals, and other nutrients from food. Even if you have a good, varied diet, alcohol may keep you from enjoying the full health benefits of that diet.

THE MALE REPRODUCTIVE SYSTEM

Scientists love acronyms—using just the first initials of words in complicated medical terms and phrases to create new words, such as *AIDS* (for "acquired immunodeficiency syndrome"). The most famous acronym has been around so long, people have probably forgotten that it *is* an acronym: *snafu* (for "situation normal all fouled up")! Speaking of snafus . . .

Here's an important acronym for those males who are considering a night of drinking: the HPG axis, for "hypothalamic-pituitary-gonadal" axis. This stands for the three key glands in the male reproductive system: the hypothalamus, the pituitary gland, and the gonads (or testicles). Frequent alcohol use damages all three glands and the hormones they produce. The results of this damage can include a lower sperm count and abnormal sperm, impotence (the inability to maintain an erection), shrunken testicles, and enlarged breasts. So forget about the myth that alcohol enhances sex!

JUST FOR WOMEN

Researchers are beginning to acknowledge that women are a unique group when it comes to drinking and the damaging effects of alcohol. For one thing, women are more vulnerable to alcohol-related health diseases than men. They develop liver and brain damage more quickly than men do—even when drinking *less* alcohol. In young women, frequent drinking also may interfere with bone growth or encourage bone loss, increasing the risk of osteoporosis, a bone disorder that causes bones to become porous and brittle.

As far as a young woman's reproductive system goes, excessive alcohol use inhibits the growth of the ovaries and the production of hormones that regulate ovulation, menstruation, and fertility. Frequent drinkers may have fertility problems later in life and suffer an increased rate of miscarriages. Drinking during pregnancy also can have profoundly damaging effects on the fetus.

ALCOHOL AND YOUR BRAIN

Perhaps nowhere else are the toxic effects of too much alcohol seen so quickly and dramatically as they are when alcohol hits the brain. Drinking can change your personality, lower your inhibitions, and encourage inappropriate, silly, or downright dangerous behavior.

Frequent alcohol use can change your brain's chemistry, erase parts of your memory, affect your ability to learn new tasks and make decisions, and lower your IQ. Two of the most disturbing alcohol-related brain problems are blackouts and alcohol psychosis.

Blackouts

A blackout, is an alcohol-induced period of amnesia, or memory loss. It is not the same as "passing out," when you are unconscious. In a blackout, which can last seconds, minutes, or hours (or in the case of serious alcoholics, days or weeks), a person appears normal (though usually drunk) to the outside world, as he or she talks and interacts with others. But he or she later has no memory of that time. The person cannot remember what was said or done, or who he or she was with, and will never be able to retrieve that memory, not even under hypnosis. This is called an "en bloc blackout," or total blackout, and is the most common form of blacking out. Sometimes, people have what are called "fragmentary blackouts," where partial memory is restored when something jogs the recollection

Scientists used to believe that only serious alcoholics had blackouts, but now experts agree that even one episode of overdrinking can cause a blackout.

It is a frightening phenomenon to the drinker, but in the best-case scenario, he or she is probably just embarrassed. At the worst-case end of the spectrum, what happens during a blackout can change one's life forever.

TEENS SPEAK

He Can't Remember a Thing

"It was so scary. You don't know what it's like until it happens to you." That's how one seventeen-year-old alcoholic describes the times he blacked out while drinking.

Now Carey goes to Alcoholics Anonymous meetings twice a week; he had been sober for a few months when he told his story. But Carey is the first to admit that he might never have done anything about his problem if he hadn't started to get blackouts.

"I used to brag about how I could hold my liquor. I was getting better and better at it; I even made money a couple of times by betting I could drink older guys under the table. My father is a heavy drinker and my uncle too, but they're not alcoholics, really; I never saw my dad drive drunk, or go to work drunk or anything like that. So I had their examples to aspire to.

"First it was beer, then vodka. By then I was drinking so much on the weekends, I had to steal money from my mother's pocketbook just to pay for the liquor. At the beginning, I felt like I was in control. After a while, I would get really drunk every time I drank. Like the vodka was finally getting to me. I wasn't a happy drunk; I was confused and upset that I wasn't in control anymore. Then I'd find myself waking up on some couch, and I couldn't remember how I got there.

"It was like some kind of time or space warp. The last thing I would remember was getting together with my friends to drink, but what happened later? I would try and try to remember, but it didn't come back. I thought I was losing my mind.

"After that, I was scared enough to talk to my minister at church about it. He put me in touch with AA."

Alcohol psychosis

Alcohol psychosis is a group of brain-related symptoms that occur after frequent, heavy drinking, often during alcohol **withdrawal**, the combination of painful and uncomfortable symptoms alcoholics feel when they stop or drastically cut back their drinking. The symptoms are similar to those of the psychiatric disorder called *schizophrenia* and can include auditory and visual **hallucinations** (seeing and hearing things that aren't there); convulsions (violent shaking of the body); delusions; phobias, which are excessive and persistent fears; violent language and/or behavior; and **delirium tremens** (commonly called "the D.T.'s"), which are intense, terrifying mental images that can happen if a person stops drinking for three to four days and are accompanied by high fevers and extremely aggressive behavior. The D.T.'s involve profound anxiety and insomnia along with convulsions. Alcohol psychosis is a serious, life-threatening condition that requires hospitalization.

WHAT YOU DON'T KNOW WILL HARM YOU
Considering alcohol's role in human diseases, smart people handle it with caution and care. However, the results show that millions of people do not follow that good example. Fortunately, you are at an age where you can make wise choices that can help you live a long and happy life.

See also: Alcohol and Violence; Binge Drinking Among Teenagers; Birth Defects and Alcohol; Effects on the Body; Sexual Behavior and Alcohol

FURTHER READING
Watson, Ronald and Adam K. Meyers, eds. *Alcohol and Heart Disease.* New York: Taylor and Francis, 2002.

■ ALCOHOL AND VIOLENCE
For the majority of people who drink, alcohol is a way to relax, to help them socialize with friends, and to put aside the pressures and tensions of life. But from time immemorial, alcohol has been associated with arguments, fights, brawls, rape, spousal and child abuse, and even suicide. In the often-quoted words of the 1993 "Special Report to the U.S. Congress on Alcohol and Health," the secretary of health and human services wrote, "Alcohol is associated with a substantial proportion of human violence, and perpetrators [those who commit crimes] are often under the influence of alcohol."

How can one substance have such contradictory effects? And what can individuals do to make sure that they are never the perpetrator or the victim of a violent alcohol-related act?

HOSTILITY AND AGGRESSION
Violence, when one person physically harms or tries to harm another person, is the most severe form of the more general behavior called *aggression*. Aggression also can be conveyed through words—hostile

remarks, insults, threats, and hurtful gossip. A person can hurt other people emotionally, or harm them by spreading lies or betraying secrets to their friends, teachers, family, or coworkers. The average person may never witness criminal violence, but he or she probably will see and hear a loud, obnoxious drunk.

DID YOU KNOW?

Youth Violence and Substance Abuse

Percentages of Youths Aged 12 to 17 Reporting Any Illicit Drug Use* or Alcohol Use in the Past Year, by the Number of Types of Violent Behaviors:** 2001

 Illicit Drug Use   Alcohol Use

* "Illicit drugs" refer to drugs that are not for legal consumption or that are used without a prescription for nonmedical reasons.

** "Violent behaviors" refer to serious fighting or attacks against others with the intent of severely hurting them.

Source: National Household Survey on Drug Abuse, Substance Abuse and Mental Health Services Administration, 2001.

To the victim, any form of aggression can be frightening. If it continues on a regular basis, it can make the victim's life miserable. Alcohol has been shown to promote aggression in all its forms. In fact, a study reported in 2000 in *Alcohol and Alcoholism* showed that aggression among men increased along with their increased blood alcohol levels (until the level got high enough to make the drinker unable to act at all). Women in this study, as in others in the past, did not show the same correlation.

Fact Or Fiction?

Cheap hard liquor is more likely to lead to violence than fine wine.

Fact: Nonsense! A glass of wine and a shot of liquor have exactly the same effect on anyone. True, a group of close friends sipping wine and sampling cheese in a neighborhood pub, with soothing music in the background, will probably not get into a fight over a misunderstood remark. But they would be just as cool and relaxed if they were sipping bourbon or scotch. On the other hand, a tired, angry loner sitting in a noisy bar ordering one drink after another may be at risk of violence, whether he is drinking the finest European wine aged in the cellars of Chateau DeFaux or the cheapest whiskey on the market.

In most cases of alcohol-related aggression and violence, one cannot put all the blame on alcohol. Very few people in happy marriages assault their spouses, even under the influence of alcohol. A law-abiding, stable citizen does not suddenly knock down and rob a passerby every time he's had "a few too many."

People who have a history of violent behavior, or who tend to be aggressive even without alcohol, may be more vulnerable to the violence-provoking effects of alcohol. Still, the statistical connection between alcohol and different forms of violence is strong enough to suggest that something about alcohol itself brings out the worst in many individuals.

WHAT IS THE MECHANISM?

Psychologists have come up with a couple of basic theories about how alcohol contributes to aggression. The most popular theory is the **disinhibition model.** This theory says that alcohol chemically blurs or deadens the parts of the brain that inhibit, or hold back, one's first impulsive reactions. In nonscientific words, when you're drunk, you lose control.

When people feel insulted or threatened, or think that someone is treating them unfairly, their first impulse may be to lash out in retaliation. But normally they control that impulse. Their better judgment tells them that a) they may have misunderstood or misinterpreted the other person, and b) it probably isn't worth fighting about, and c) in any case, if they fight, they might get hurt.

Any time two people strongly disagree, the disagreement has the potential to become nasty, or even violent. Fighting is usually the "easy" way out. It is harder and more challenging to find a delicate compromise, to think of a less offensive way of making a point or to simply "agree to disagree." Unfortunately, alcohol makes that even harder to achieve, by numbing a drinker's mental faculties.

If this theory is true, anyone has the potential to become aggressive under the influence of alcohol when faced with provocation or threats. But the people most at risk are those who are prone to violence even when sober.

Some researchers have recently tried to figure out the precise mechanism behind disinhibition. For example, according to psychologist James W. Kalat, in the 2001 book *Biological Psychology*, alcohol may reduce the activity of serotonin, a chemical messenger in the brain that is believed to act as an inhibitor. Other key brain chemicals involved in behavior and mood, such as dopamine, may also be disrupted by alcohol.

The second theory is called **alcohol expectancy.** This theory claims that in some cultures, people believe that alcohol all by itself can turn a drinker violent. When people with that notion drink, they almost expect to get into fights. In some laboratory studies, people became more aggressive after drinking a nonalcoholic beverage that they *believed* was alcohol. Similarly, some criminals say they use alcohol to overcome their fears and inhibitions before committing a violent crime. They too believe in the equation: Alcohol means aggression. These expectations may encourage the behavior.

These theories are interesting, but they may not tell the full story. Sometimes, an emotional problem makes people act in a hostile and aggressive manner, *and* the same problem leads them to abuse alcohol as an escape. In those cases, it is not accurate to say that alcohol abuse caused the violence; they are both the result of the *underlying* emotional cause.

There may be another reason to take the statistics about alcohol and crime with a grain of salt. Common sense tells us that criminals under the influence of alcohol may not be careful about hiding their tracks; that probably makes it easier for the police to find them. Because sober criminals may be more likely to escape detection, they do not wind up in the statistics. In other words, it may *look* as if all the perpetrators are drinking, because the ones who don't drink are not caught.

There is also a feedback effect between violence and alcohol. People who have been victimized by violence are more likely to abuse alcohol; under the influence, they may in turn commit violence against other people. This can happen within families, as each new generation repeats the patterns learned from the previous one.

VIOLENT CRIMES

In a 1997 report, the National Institute on Alcohol Abuse and Alcoholism reported that a huge percentage of murderers were drinking at the time of their crimes—as many as 86 percent of them in some areas. Up to 37 percent of those committing assault also had been drinking. Most other categories of crime showed similar high correlations with alcohol, including sexual assault and rape. The numbers are highest for spousal abuse: More than 60 percent of violence between spouses or partners involves alcohol.

Robbery also gets into the picture. Robbers need a clear head to plan and carry out their crimes, yet, according to a 2001 article in *Alcohol Research and Health,* nearly one third of the people jailed for robbery say they had been drinking at the time of the crime. The article also reported that a 1998 survey of violent offenders found that 38 percent of those in state prisons, 41 percent of those in local jails, and 41 percent of those on probation "reported that they had been using alcohol when they committed their offenses."

You may be saying to yourself, "This is not *me.* I would never attack another person, no matter how much alcohol I drink." That may be true, yet the issue may still affect you more than you think, because a large percentage of the *victims* of violent crimes were also drinking when the crimes were committed.

Without intending to, people can sometimes innocently provoke a violent attack. The recipe for violence often is: violent tendencies (on the part of the aggressor), too much alcohol, and a word or gesture (by the victim) that is misinterpreted as a provocation.

People under the influence of alcohol are not likely to be tactful. They may say or do things, with no malicious intent, that they would never say or do when sober. As they continue to dig themselves into a hole, they may be too drunk to notice the facial expressions and body language of others that should be flashing the warning: "Change the subject, sit down, stop waving your arms in the air." None of this excuses the person who commits a violent act, but it does suggest that being even mildly intoxicated can sometimes be quite dangerous even for a nonviolent individual.

Finally, when you are drunk, you are an easy target for criminals. For example, you may exercise poor judgment while alone in an isolated area. And when danger approaches, you may not be able to talk your way out of it or, if need be, to run away.

SEXUAL ASSAULT AND RAPE

Every major study on the subject of rape and sexual assault shows a strong correlation between these crimes and alcohol. Very often, both the perpetrator and the victim had been drinking when the crime took place.

Apart from the general link between alcohol and violence, additional factors are involved in sexual crimes. The male perpetrator may believe that alcohol enhances his sexual abilities. In fact, studies have shown that it does the opposite; it is generally harder for a man to perform sexually after drinking more than a minimum amount.

The perpetrator may also believe in some old-fashioned myths about women and alcohol, which sensible people have long ago discarded. For example, he may believe that "nice" women do not drink in public, so any woman who does so is probably available for sex. He may assume that a woman who agrees to drink with him is giving him license to take sexual advantage of her. Or he may honestly misinterpret her words and behavior—alcohol can prevent people from "reading" the complicated clues and hidden messages that govern sexual behavior.

Rapists often "excuse" their behavior by blaming alcohol, and they may even drink in advance in order to give themselves an excuse. They also may knowingly exploit the fact that women get intoxicated on smaller amounts of alcohol and deliberately get women to drink too much.

The female victim may also allow alcohol to cloud her judgment. Most women become intoxicated much sooner after drinking the same amount of alcohol as a man. Their ability to communicate their desires, including the decision not to engage in sexual behavior, may be impaired. And when the attack begins, women may not have all the mental and physical resources they need to fend it off.

CHILD ABUSE

Some of the saddest cases of alcohol-related violence involve child abuse. This can include incest, usually committed by fathers, or physical abuse, which mothers are as likely to commit as fathers.

The National Center on Addiction and Substance Abuse at Columbia University issued some frightening figures in a 1999 report. Children whose parents abuse alcohol and other drugs are 2.7 times more likely to physically abuse their children. Most child welfare and court professionals told the researchers that alcohol and other drugs caused, or contributed to, more than half of all cases of physical abuse. It should be noted, however, that scientific surveys of the evidence do not always show that alcohol is the cause of violent child abuse.

When a parent is drunk, any kind of normal childhood behavior can trigger a violent response. Older kids may learn to avoid their parents or to withdraw emotionally. Younger kids, however, may simply be unable to keep themselves from crying, disobeying, or somehow annoying their parents.

Alcohol is estimated to be involved in close to half of all reported cases of incest. In addition, even parents who do not themselves abuse their children may, if they abuse alcohol, be unable to prevent other adults, sometimes alcohol abusers themselves, from harming their children.

TEENS SPEAK

I Still Cry When I Remember

Seth's mother is now in recovery, and they get along fine when she comes to visit. But he still gets very emotional when he lets himself think of the period last year when she really cracked.

"It's not like we didn't know she was an alcoholic. I was thirteen years old then, but even my younger brother Jordan understood that Mom had a problem with booze. When she would drink, in the afternoons before Dad came home, we used to steer clear. Any little thing would tick her off and she'd start yelling and hitting us—not hard, just to get us away from her. But she would always come in to apologize before we went to bed.

"Then Mom and Dad started to fight. He used to drink a little too, and he'd call her names, like say she was a lousy mother and things. She'd scream at him, and sometimes they threw punches. Then he would leave and slam the door.

"Then one time last year, she took a real swing at Jordan, and he fell against the edge of the table. He started screaming, and I saw he had a big gash right under his eye. Mom told me to call 911, but she was too drunk to come with the ambulance; they had to call Dad.

"In the end Jordan had three stitches; he'll probably always have this big scar.

"I was so mad at Mom at first, but when we came home she fell all over us crying, and apologized a million times. It was really pathetic; I just hated her and wouldn't let her off the hook. But now I understand better; it was really the liquor talking, not Mom. Since she went sober we get along much better."

SPOUSAL ABUSE

Of all violent crimes, spousal abuse is the one most associated with alcohol. A study of 2,000 American couples in 1993 showed that domestic violence rates are *15 times* higher in households where husbands are often drunk than in households where the husbands are never drunk.

Broader studies show that between 60 and 70 percent of spousal violence cases involve alcohol. Usually, both partners have been drinking. Clearly, these incidents involve many other issues apart from just alcohol. Sometimes, when alcohol abuse itself is a major subject of contention between the partners, one partner taking a single drink can trigger a violent confrontation.

Cultural approval of violence is the strongest factor that determines whether or not an argument between spouses or partners may escalate to violence. In other words, if a man believes that his religion, ethnic group, or community grants him a right to dominate his partner or to use force, he may well act on that belief. On the other hand, if he believes spousal abuse will be met with disapproval in his social circles, he is less likely to use that type of force.

In many cases of spousal violence, the female partner is involved in violent behavior as well as the male, and she may have had as much to drink. However, women are more likely than men to suffer moderate or severe physical violence and harm, even in cases where they initiated the violence.

SELF-MUTILATION

Self-mutilation, or deliberate self-harm, is a serious emotional disorder that affects many teenagers, more often girls than boys. It may include hitting, cutting or burning one's skin, pulling one's hair, and even taking poison. The individual does not want to do any lasting harm, but he or she cannot control the impulse. No one knows why some kids behave this way, but some therapists believe they are trying to cover up emotional pain with physical pain.

Kids who mutilate themselves also may abuse alcohol or other drugs. In some cases, alcohol or drug use can worsen the problem by contributing to feelings of low self-esteem and hopelessness.

SUICIDE

About 25,000–30,000 Americans kill themselves every year, and many thousands more attempt suicide. The National Center for Substance Abuse Prevention reported in 1995 that alcohol seems to be one of the contributing factors in many of these sad cases. The center reported studies showing that more than one third of suicide victims had positive BAL, or blood alcohol levels, the percentage of alcohol in a person's bloodstream at any one time, and almost one quarter had BALs of .1 or higher, which is considered intoxication in every state. Even worse, alcohol is particularly associated with unplanned, impulsive suicides rather than with premeditated acts. Because alcohol can reduce inhibitions, impair judgment, and make depression worse, any one of those effects could push a suicidal person over the edge.

In 2002, the National Household Survey on Drug Abuse found that kids aged 12 to 17 are more than twice as likely to be at risk for suicide if they drink alcohol. (The figure rises to three times as likely for kids who use illegal drugs, apart from marijuana.)

The lesson is clear. Anyone unhappy enough to have considered ending his or her life must be very careful about choosing whether, where, when, and with whom to drink.

Q & A

Question: How common is suicide among kids? Isn't it really an adult problem?

Answer: Unfortunately, suicide is common among adolescents in the United States. It is the fourth leading cause of death for kids aged 10 to 14 and the third leading cause of death in the 15 to 25 age group. If you are depressed about your problems and feel like ending it all, why not give yourself another chance? Instead of picking up a bottle, pick up the phone and get help—from a friend, relative, teacher, doctor, or hot line.

A COMMON PROBLEM

Whatever the cause-and-effect relationship may be, alcohol is associated with violence of many different kinds. Anyone who drinks, or plans to drink, should keep this relationship in mind. If an individual, a particular situation, or a setting has the potential for violence, sensible people will stay away from that next drink—or any drink at all.

See also: Drinking on College Campuses; Sexual Behavior and Alcohol

FURTHER READING

Lawrence A. Greenfield. *Alcohol and Crime: An Analysis of National Data on the Prevalence of Alcohol Involvement in Crime.* Washington D.C.: Bureau of Justice Statistics, 1998.

Robert Nash Parker. *Alcohol and Crime: A Deadly Combination of Two American Traditions.* Albany, NY: State University of New York Press, 1995.

■ ALCOHOLISM, CAUSES OF

Despite decades of research and the efforts of many scientists, no one has discovered a single, definitive cause of alcoholism, also known as the addiction to alcohol, or the physical and emotional dependency on alcohol. In fact, so many theories about alcoholism have evolved over the last two centuries that when noted alcohol scholar E. M. Jellinek wrote his famous 1960 book *The Disease Concept of Alcoholism*, he identified more than 200 theories and definitions of alcoholism!

Historical theories of alcoholism include the moral and temperance models of the 19th and early 20th centuries. In the 1930s, the "alcoholism as a disease" concept became popular and is still the prevailing theory in many recovery movements. Less popular, but equally important, are theories that attempt to factor in the unique personality, social, cultural, or behavioral characteristics of alcoholics.

Starting in the 1970s, scientists who had long suspected a biological cause of alcohol abuse began studying **alcoholics** for genetic (physical traits inherited from parents) and biochemical similarities. By the end of the twentieth century, researchers had indeed found a strong biological component to alcoholism.

Nevertheless, all experts agree that social, cultural, and emotional factors play a major role in alcohol abuse as well. For example, kids who grow up in communities or social groups where getting drunk is acceptable may eventually become alcoholics, even if none of them seem to have biological tendencies in that direction. In other words, alcoholism has multiple causes.

Here is a brief look at some of the more popular theories about the cause of alcoholism.

THE MORALITY AND TEMPERANCE THEORIES

The **morality theory** of alcoholism places the blame squarely on the individual. Put simply, the theory proposes that responsible people with strong moral fiber do not drink; weak-willed people with no spiritual backbone *do* drink—in fact, they drink too much and get in a lot of trouble. This was a popular theory in the eighteenth and nineteenth centuries. While it sounds puritanical and old-fashioned, the idea that alcoholics are deviant people with no willpower is one that still persists in many people's views today.

The **temperance movement** that began in the late eighteenth century and thrived in the nineteenth had its own theory of alcoholism. It shifted the blame for alcohol abuse from the individual to alcohol itself. While at first the movement favored moderate drinking, over time it began to view alcohol as an inherently dangerous substance that no one could drink safely in any amount.

The temperance movement in the United States culminated in 1919 in the passage of the Eighteenth Amendment to the U.S. Constitution, which prohibited the manufacture and sale of alcohol. **Prohibition** (which *prohibited* the sale of alcoholic beverages), lasted for 14 years. Though the law did indeed cause a major reduction in drinking and alcohol abuse, especially outside urban areas, it also generated some major problems of its own. Public opinion turned against Prohibition, and in 1933 the Twenty-first Amendment put an end to the experiment.

THE DISEASE THEORY

Two years after Prohibition ended in 1933, the **Alcoholics Anonymous** (A.A.) program began, and A.A. groups sprang up across the United States. Proponents of the A.A. program of recovery claimed that alcoholism was a progressive, incurable, and potentially fatal disease to which a certain small group of individuals—alcoholics—were uniquely susceptible. According to the **disease theory**, alcoholics (who can never drink safely) are physically different from nonalcoholics (who can drink safely). Since alcoholism has no cure, the **recovering alcoholic** must practice lifelong sobriety: He or she must never drink again.

The disease theory of alcoholism was embraced strongly by alcoholics and nonalcoholics alike, as well as by the liquor industry and the medical community. Today, it is still a powerful concept in recovery programs and among physicians and substance abuse counselors. Though a small but vocal group believe that alcoholics can learn to drink moderately and safely, most experts encourage alcohol abusers to give up drinking entirely.

THE PERSONALITY, SOCIOCULTURAL, AND BEHAVIORAL THEORIES

Personality theories of alcoholism have their roots in psychoanalysis, a method of investigating mental processes by means of confronting repressed thoughts. In the 1940s and 1950s, psychiatrists proposed several theories about alcoholics. One suggested that alcoholics had never progressed beyond some critical stage in their personality development, usually the "oral stage," the primary focus of the first months of a baby's life when pleasure derives from things in the mouth. Other theories considered alcoholics to have low self-esteem or to suffer from sex-role or sexual identity conflicts. These theories are not widely accepted today.

Psychologists, social workers, and substance abuse counselors have long identified various social and cultural causes of alcohol abuse. They believe that people who belong to social circles where heavy drinking is the norm (such as various professions or ethnic groups), or who live in places where alcohol is available and cheap or in subcultures that associate alcohol with drunkenness, are more likely to abuse the beverage, whatever their underlying personalities. They also believe people can become dependent on alcohol due to financial or emotional stress, poor coping skills, and susceptibility to peer pressure.

The behavioral theory considers alcoholism to be a learned behavior. **Conditioning** by the family and the community, reinforced by peers and even by liquor advertising can teach people unhealthy behavior patterns, to the extent that the first drink, or even the sight of a bar on a street, kicks off a chain of events leading to intoxication. Treatment usually involves **counterconditioning**, or behavioral therapy, in which the alcoholic learns new, healthier ways of responding to the stimulus of alcohol.

Fact Or Fiction?

Three million American teens are alcoholics.

Fact: Yes. The National Institute of Alcoholism and Alcohol Abuse reported in 2000 that nearly three million young people between the ages of 14 and 17 "are regular drinkers with a serious alcohol problem." Typically, their first experience of alcohol intoxication occurs in the early to mid-teens. Historically, teenage boys drank more alcohol than teenage girls, but in recent years the gap between the genders has almost disappeared.

BIOLOGICAL THEORIES:
HEREDITY, GENETICS, AND BIOCHEMISTRY

For centuries, medical experts and lay people alike have observed that alcohol abuse runs in families and seems to be passed down from one generation to the next. That fact has become a given. The real question is: Why? The challenge to researchers is figuring out how to separate "nature from nurture" in the development of family-related alcoholism. In other words, are children of alcoholics at a higher risk for alcoholism because they inherited a gene that makes it difficult to handle alcohol ("nature"), or do they learn alcoholic behaviors from observing their parents as they grow up ("nurture")?

In recent decades, scientists have tried to discover a possible genetic link to alcoholism by looking at twins and at children adopted into or out of alcoholic families.

Heredity: twin and adoption studies

A famous 1960s study of the drinking patterns of more than 900 twins in Finland sparked a generation of similar research projects in the United States. Identical (or monozygotic) twins share the same genes. Fraternal (or dizygotic) twins share no more genes than other brothers and sisters. Studies have consistently found that identical twins are significantly more likely to *both* be alcoholic (when one is alcoholic) than are nonidentical twins (when one is alcoholic). These studies seem to support a strong genetic link to alcoholism—the "nature" part of the question, though they generally do not look at environmental factors ("nurture") that might be at work as well.

Adoption studies *have* looked at both sides of the question. Large-scale adoption studies done in the late 1970s and the 1980s compared adopted male children who had at least one alcoholic biological parent to adopted males who had no biological family history of alcohol abuse. The adopted children whose biological parents were alcoholic were four times more likely to become alcoholic themselves, even when they were raised in nonalcoholic adoptive families.

Furthermore, the studies showed that adopted children from non-alcoholic biological families had significantly lower rates of alcoholism, even when they grew up with alcoholic foster or adoptive parents. Taken together, the studies suggest that genetic makeup is a much stronger influence than environment.

Q & A

Question: My big sister was lecturing me about not drinking. She says that since my parents are alcoholics and because I'm a boy, I could become an alcoholic too. Is that true?

Answer: Between 20 and 25 percent of the sons and brothers of alcoholics become alcoholics themselves. In contrast, only 5 percent of the daughters and sisters of alcoholics become alcoholics. However, whether male or female, child or sibling, those with a genetic tendency for alcoholism are more likely to begin abusing alcohol at a younger age than their peers, become alcoholic sooner, and have a more severe form of alcoholism. More reasons, if you come from a family with a history of alcohol abuse, to think long and hard before picking up that first drink.

Genetics and biochemistry

In the 1990s, the National Institute of Alcohol Abuse and Alcoholism (NIAAA) and the Collaborative Study on the Genetics of Alcoholism (COGA) launched a long-term study to identify the actual genes that may cause alcoholism. Researchers are analyzing the genetic makeup of 1,000 individuals from families with a history of alcoholism. To date, scientists have identified a possible strong genetic link to increased alcohol **dependence** on chromosomes 1 and 7, and a more modest link for dependence on chromosome 2.

Researchers have also identified genetic variations that may work to *prevent* alcoholism. These variations are in the genes that produce enzymes that speed up the body's metabolism, or breaking down process, of alcohol. When the body breaks down alcohol quickly, a large amount of the toxic chemical **acetaldehyde** is released, making the drinker feel sick and "flushed." In general, people who suffer this reaction avoid alcohol, or drink very little. For example, there is a relatively low rate of alcoholism among East Asians, many of whom have the genes that cause them to experience the flushing reaction when they drink even a small amount of alcohol (as reported by the NIAAA in 1998). The unpleasant sensations more than balance out the "high" they may get from alcohol.

The NIAAA and COGA researchers found that individuals from alcoholic families who did *not* become alcohol abusers themselves had these protective genes. These people appear to have a built-in genetic protection against abusing alcohol.

Acetaldehyde also figures prominently in some studies linking brain chemistry and alcoholism. For instance, acetaldehyde combines with other chemicals in the brain to produce compounds called TIQs. TIQs chemically resemble morphine, a powerfully addictive opiate. This process may account for the "craving" for alcohol that many alcohol abusers experience.

Thus, a single byproduct of alcohol can have opposite effects on different people. For those who break down alcohol quickly, high levels of acetaldehyde produce unpleasant symptoms that turn them off alcohol. For those who break down alcohol gradually, the same chemical helps create powerful cravings for the beverage.

Alcohol also appears to increase or decrease levels of certain brain chemicals, notably serotonin, a complex chemical in the brain that transmits nerve signals. An imbalance in serotonin levels has been linked to depression; when levels are restored, a feeling of well-being seems to result. To the extent that alcohol may increase serotonin levels, some drinkers may be unwittingly "medicating themselves" when they drink.

Some alcoholics show imbalances in brain chemistry, according to George F. Koob, head of an NIAAA research program on the microbiology of alcoholism. Koob said in April, 2003, that some alcoholics may have a hyperactive stress system, and may be using alcohol just "to feel normal." However it is not clear whether the imbalance causes alcoholism or vice versa.

GENETICS—AND EVERYTHING ELSE

Most experts now agree that genetics plays a major role in the development of alcoholism. They generally estimate that between 40 and 60 percent of the risk for alcoholism is genetic. But genetics is not the only cause. Ongoing research should clarify the relative role of the other factors, including social and psychological problems and the influence of subcultures and peer groups.

See also: Alcohol Abuse, the Risks of; Alcohol and Violence; Alcohol, History of; Drinking and Drugs; Recovery and Treatment; Underage Drinking

FURTHER READING

William F. Asbury and Katherine Ketcham. *Beyond the Influence: Understanding and Defeating Alcoholism.* New York: Bantam Books, 2000.

Ronald Marshall. *Alcoholism: Genetic Culpability or Social Irresponsibility.* Lanham, MD: University Press of America, 2001.

■ BINGE DRINKING AMONG TEENAGERS

Not all people who study alcohol abuse use the term *binge drinking* the same way. However, the definition used by the National Household Survey on Drug Abuse (NHSDA) is a good place to start.

NHSDA defines binge drinking as consuming "five or more drinks on the same occasion on at least 1 day in the past 30 days. By 'occasion' is meant at the same time or within a couple of hours of each other." To the NHSDA, a "drink" is a 1.5-ounce shot of 80-proof liquor, a 12-ounce bottle of regular beer, or a 5-ounce glass of wine.

WHAT IS BINGE DRINKING?

Alcohol can intoxicate some people after one or two drinks. Teenagers who have never had alcohol may experience that the first time they drink. Even many adults, if they only drink on special occasions, can get tipsy after just a couple of drinks.

Other people find it harder to get drunk and feel they have to work at it. You may ask: Does anybody really *try* to get drunk? According to data compiled in 2002 by Monitoring the Future, a project of the National Institute on Drug Abuse, most teenagers *don't*—four out of five have not been drunk lately. Also, although more than 40 percent of high school kids have been drunk at least once, they usually don't repeat the experience.

Unfortunately, however, some teenagers do make an effort to get drunk, and they do it time after time. Those people are binge drinkers—they have frequent episodes of drinking too much. This is the most widespread form of alcohol abuse among young Americans. According to the Youth Risk Behavior Surveillance System, some 30 percent of high school students in 2001 reported binge drinking in the previous month.

Some kids may binge once, suffer harmful or even disastrous consequences, and never do it again. Some other teens, usually older, can manage to have four or five drinks once in a while without causing serious harm to themselves or others and without becoming alcohol dependent. Some people would call them binge drinkers; others would not. But the experts agree that far too many teenagers in America have a serious problem with binge drinking. Thousands of kids are bingeing, and they are putting their lives and futures at risk.

The Harvard School of Public Health limits the term "binge drinker" to those who have had five or more drinks on one occasion in the past *two weeks* rather than 30 days. They use the five-drink cutoff point for men but lower it to four drinks for women, since women are more likely to become intoxicated, and suffer physical harm, with less alcohol. Using different standards makes it difficult to compare the results of different surveys.

The Higher Education Center for Alcohol and Other Drug Prevention, an agency of the U.S. Department of Education, deals with the very real problem of alcohol abuse on college campuses. In 2000, the center said that five drinks should not always be considered a binge. A better definition, it said, would take into account the drinker's body weight, as well as how fast he or she drinks and how much food he or she eats while drinking. All those factors change the impact of alcohol on the body and brain. College officials, the center said, found that students were dismissing messages against alcohol abuse, since they believed the definitions were unrealistic.

Fact Or Fiction?

People who graduate from college drink more than other Americans.

Fact: The above statement is a half-truth. According to the National Household Survey of Drug Abuse, almost two-thirds of all college graduates drink, compared with only one-third of people age 18 or older who never finished high school. However, the higher the level of formal education people have, the more likely they are to be moderate in their drinking habits. As a result, alcohol abuse, including bingeing, is less common among college graduates than among any other group.

However they define the term, all these agencies find it useful to distinguish binge drinkers from heavy drinkers and **alcoholics.** "Bingers" do not necessarily progress to heavy drinking (usually defined as bingeing several times a month), and they may never feel the physical or emotional cravings that dominate the lives of alcoholics.

Teenage drinkers should not take too much comfort in this distinction. Anyone who deliberately drinks to the point of intoxication, even on just an occasional basis, is engaging in binge drinking, with all its risks. It is especially worrisome if he or she intends to do so again in the future.

Sometimes bingeing is obvious. Teenagers often tell therapists and counselors about "drinking games," in which one participant pours alcohol into another person's mouth directly from a bottle or through a funnel, in which teens take turns drinking directly from a beer keg, or in which kids swallow "Jell-O shots." These are obvious examples of binge drinking.

But binge drinking also occurs when a few young friends get into the habit of gathering every Sunday to watch an afternoon of ball games and drink one light beer after another until some or all of them are drunk. And of course, anyone who blacks out during drinking and cannot remember later some or all of what happened is bingeing dangerously.

HOW COMMON IS BINGEING?

Until experts agree on a definition, any numbers must be considered estimates. But the best estimates issued by government agencies offer both good and bad news. The good news is that teenage bingeing has declined in the last few years, and has declined even more as compared with 20 years ago. The bad news is, bingeing is still a major problem.

Monitoring the Future has some of the best data for binge drinking, which they also call heavy episodic drinking and which they define as five drinks or more in the past two weeks. They report that the practice had declined among 12th graders from 41 percent in 1983 to 28 percent in 1992. After rising for a while in the 1990s, it began declining again, and fell to 28.6 percent in 2002.

In addition, more 12th graders today seem to understand the risks involved in bingeing. In 1982, 36 percent believed that drinking heavily once or twice each weekend carried a "great risk"; the number rose to 49 percent in 1992. In 2002, 42 percent believed so, as did more than half of eighth and 10th graders.

Among eighth graders, 12.4 percent engaged in binge drinking in 2002, marking the third year of decline from a 15.2 percent high in 1999. For 10th graders, the figures were 22.4 percent in 2002, compared with 25.6 percent in 1999. For both grades, however, only slightly fewer kids had engaged in heavy episodic drinking in 2002 than ten years before.

Monitoring the Future reported figures for binge drinking among various subgroups within the grades. In 2002, for eighth graders, the gender breakdown was 13.7 percent for boys and 12.4 for girls. The racial breakdown was 17.6 percent for Hispanic Americans, 9.0 percent for African Americans, and 13.8 percent for Caucasians. Only 11.2 percent of those who planned to complete four years of college binged, as compared with 29.6 percent of the others.

The greatest contrasts involved the parents' education level. Twenty-one percent of the eighth graders whose parents did not complete high school binged, while only 8.1 percent of those whose parents attended graduate school did so. For 10th and 12th graders, the gender and racial breakdowns were similar, but the effect of parents' education and kids' college plans became much less important.

For Americans as a whole, binge drinking seems to peak at age 21 and declines as the age group advances. This suggests that the majority of people who binge as kids "outgrow" the experience. Unfortunately, some get stuck along the way, with serious consequences.

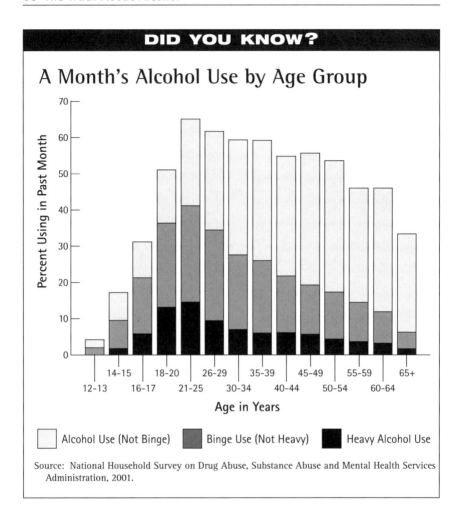

DID YOU KNOW?

A Month's Alcohol Use by Age Group

Percent Using in Past Month (y-axis, 0 to 70)

Age in Years (x-axis): 12-13, 14-15, 16-17, 18-20, 21-25, 26-29, 30-34, 35-39, 40-44, 45-49, 50-54, 55-59, 60-64, 65+

Legend:
☐ Alcohol Use (Not Binge) ▨ Binge Use (Not Heavy) ■ Heavy Alcohol Use

Source: National Household Survey on Drug Abuse, Substance Abuse and Mental Health Services Administration, 2001.

RISKS

The American Psychological Association reported in 2001 that according to the latest evidence, heavy drinking by teens might do more damage to their nervous systems than had been thought. According to these studies, the human brain continues to develop until the age of 21. As a result, "teens who binge drink may do damage to their memory and learning abilities by severely hampering the development of the hippocampus." (This small but important part of the brain has a major role in storing memories and regulating motivation.)

Of course, most of the behavioral risks that pertain to alcohol abuse apply to binge drinking. Bingers are responsible for a large proportion of DWI motor vehicle accidents involving teens. The more frequent and intense the binges, the more drinkers are likely to also engage in risky sex, injure themselves, and be victims of violent crimes. The outward physical effects of bingeing, such as extreme intoxication or passing out in public, also ensure that teenage bingers have a good chance of getting in trouble with the law.

Binge drinking can also sometimes lead to alcohol **dependency**. It is not true, as some people mistakenly believe, that you can't become an alcoholic if you drink only on weekends. Several studies have found that high school binge drinkers are very likely to binge drink in college as well, according to a 1995 report from the National Institute of Alcohol Abuse and Alcoholism. This type of behavior pattern, which lasts for several years, can become hard to break, even though high school and college bingers often do not believe they are problem drinkers.

SECONDHAND EFFECTS OF BINGEING

Teenagers are notorious for thinking they are "immortal." Even when they fully understand the dangers of risky behavior, they sometimes find it hard to believe that "it could happen to me." If you are one of those teens, then at least consider the real risk that if you binge, you may harm other people. Innocent bystanders who do not voluntarily assume the risk often become the victims.

Motor vehicle accidents do the most damage, but binge drinking impacts other secondhand victims too. A report released in 1998 by the College Alcohol Study of the Harvard School of Public Health stated that four out of five on-campus students who were not binge drinkers had experienced at least one second-hand effect of bingeing, including assault, unwanted sexual advances, property damage, and having sleep or study disturbed.

LEARN THE FACTS

Despite attempts to educate kids to the dangers of binge drinking, teenage bingeing remains a serious problem in the United States. Kids need to learn the facts in order to be able to make the intelligent choice when the situation arises.

See also: Alcohol Abuse, The Risks of; Drinking on College Campuses

FURTHER READING
Margaret O. Hyde, John F. Setaro. *Alcohol 101: An Overview for Teens*. Bookfield, CT: Twenty-first Century, 1999.
Gail B. Stewart. *Teen Alcoholics*. San Diego, CA: Lucent, 2000.
James D. Torr, ed. *Alcoholism*. San Diego, CA: Greenhaven, 2000.

■ BIRTH DEFECTS AND ALCOHOL

A birth defect is a health problem that develops while the baby is forming inside the mother. The defect may be inherited or acquired. One of the leading causes of birth defects, mental retardation, and developmental disabilities in children is also 100 percent preventable—drinking during pregnancy. Yet every year, one in thirty pregnant women indulges in risk drinking that may damage her baby.

Risk drinking is defined as seven or more drinks per week (also called frequent drinking or heavy drinking, or five or more drinks on one occasion (called binge drinking). Another one in seven women of childbearing age, who is pregnant but not aware of it, also engages in risk drinking.

The range of alcohol-related birth defects and disabilities runs the spectrum from mild learning and social problems to profound retardation. The most severe form of alcohol-related disorder is **fetal alcohol syndrome**, commonly known as FAS.

FETAL ALCOHOL SYNDROME

When a pregnant mother drinks, the alcohol in her bloodstream easily crosses the placenta, an organ in most mammals that connects the developing fetus to the mother's uterus and enters her baby's system through the umbilical cord. While scientists are still not sure exactly how alcohol damages a baby in utero (that is, in the mother's uterus or womb), they do know that FAS, the severest form of alcohol-related birth defects, is most frequently associated with frequent or heavy drinking, binge drinking, and alcoholism.

FAS is actually a group of alcohol-related birth abnormalities that primarily affect three areas: the face, the brain, and growth.

Facial abnormalities

Many children with FAS have a distinctive facial appearance, which may include any of the following: a small head; widely spaced eyes with epicanthic folds (an elongation of the fold in the upper eyelids); a low nasal bridge and flat midface; a short nose; minor ear abnormalities; a thin upper lip; or a narrowed jaw. These facial abnormalities occur during the first trimester (first three months) of pregnancy.

Facial, organ, and bone damage generally happen because of drinking during the first trimester of pregnancy. During the third and fourth week of this trimester, the embryo's arms, central nervous system, eyes, heart, and legs are developing and are especially vulnerable to damage.

Brain abnormalities

FAS-related brain and central nervous system abnormalities can occur throughout pregnancy and may include: moderate to severe mental retardation; low IQ; developmental delays; speech and language delays; behavior disorders; and poor learning, memory, and problem-solving skills.

The brain of the unborn child develops throughout pregnancy, during all three trimesters, so brain damage related to alcohol can happen at any time during pregnancy.

Growth abnormalities

Infants born with FAS are often significantly underweight and smaller than other newborns, putting them at greater risk for lung and heart failure, and for viral and bacterial infections during the newborn period. They also may have skeletal abnormalities, organ defects, and hearing problems. As children, they are generally smaller in stature and slower to grow than unaffected children and may have poor coordination and muscle control. These FAS-related growth effects can occur throughout pregnancy. However, alcohol-related low birth weight and smaller-than-average size are most associated with drinking during the *third* trimester (last three months) of pregnancy.

Q & A

Question: My friend told me it's okay to drink when I'm pregnant. What amount of alcohol is safe to drink?

Answer: *No* amount of alcohol is safe to drink during pregnancy—or if you are trying to *get* pregnant, since many women do not know that they are pregnant for three to eight weeks after conception. While frequent or heavy drinking, alcoholic drinking, and binge drinking are most associated with severe damage to the unborn child, any alcohol consumed increases the chances of a child being born with physical, learning, and behavioral problems. Despite what some people believe, there is no "safe time" to drink during pregnancy.

Prevalence of FAS

Scientists do not know the exact prevalence of FAS. ("Prevalence" refers to the percentage of a population affected by a disease or disorder at a given time.) Prevalence rates found vary by type of research study done and by populations studied. Studies by the Centers for Disease Control and Prevention (CDC) in the 1990s have found FAS prevalence rates between 0.2 and 1.5 per 1,000 live births in different areas of the country. Rates as high as three per 1,000 live births have been found among some populations. These figures roughly translate to several thousand babies born in the United States with FAS each year.

Fact Or Fiction?

Any drinking during pregnancy causes birth defects.

Fact: The truth is, some women can drink during a pregnancy and have healthy babies; but many other women and their babies are vulnerable to alcohol's toxic effects, even when they drink only small quantities. And this is good news for the many healthy babies born to mothers who drink during pregnancy. But it is bad news for maternal and child health care advocates who work hard to educate young women about the dangers of drinking during pregnancy. Scientists do not know why this is true, and they cannot predict which women and babies are most susceptible. The bottom line is: The only sure way to protect your baby from alcohol-related birth defects is not to drink.

OTHER ALCOHOL-RELATED BIRTH DISORDERS

Although full-blown FAS is a profoundly damaging disorder, it is relatively rare. However, other very serious alcohol-related birth disorders occur with greater frequency.

Many children diagnosed with FAS have a distinctly less severe form of the condition. Other children exposed to their mothers' drinking during pregnancy have some (but not all) of the symptoms of FAS. In the past, scientists used the general term "fetal alcohol effects" (FAE) to describe the FAS-like disorders of both groups of children. Currently, most researchers use two other terms, which more clearly define FAE: alcohol-related neurodevelopmental disorder (ARND) and alcohol-related birth defects (ARBD).

ARND refers to the mental, learning, and behavioral problems experienced by a child exposed to a mother's alcohol use during pregnancy. Symptoms include poor academic performance; impaired mathematical skills; alcohol-related attention deficit hyperactivity disorder (ADHD); other attention, judgment, and impulse disorders; memory impairment; and poor emotional control.

ARBD is used to describe alcohol-caused physical defects and includes deformities of the face, skull, skeleton, and auditory system, as well as defects in the heart, kidneys, and other organs.

The prevalence of ARND and ARBD (together often called FAE) is far greater than FAS but more difficult to estimate because the disorders are frequently harder to diagnose as alcohol-related.

THE COSTS OF FAS AND FAE

FAS and FAE are incurable disorders that affect a child physically, intellectually, emotionally, and behaviorally throughout his or her life. The impact on the child's family, which invariably needs much outside support, is also huge and lasts a lifetime. These kinds of costs are immeasurable.

The *economic* costs associated with FAS and FAE are estimated at nearly $3 billion a year. The average lifetime cost of treating one person with FAS or FAE is $3 million and includes monies spent for counseling; the criminal justice, prison, and welfare systems; family outreach programs; health care; and special education.

HELP SPREAD THE WORD

Fortunately, the message has gotten out to most people: Drinking during pregnancy can have devastating consequences for the woman and for her child. Birth defects are always heart breaking; when they could have been prevented, they are tragic. Teens can and should do their part to spread the word and help eliminate FAS from their society.

See also: Alcohol and Disease; Alcoholism, Causes of; Binge Drinking Among Teenagers; Sexual Behavior and Alcohol

FURTHER READING
Liz Kulp. *The Best I Can Be: Living with Fetal Alcohol Syndrome Effects*. Brooklyn Park, MN: Better Endings New Beginnings, 2000.
Amy Nevitt. *Fetal Alcohol Syndrome*. New York: Rosen Publishing Group, 1996.

■ CAUSES OF ALCOHOLISM

See: Alcoholism, Causes of

■ CHILDREN AND ALCOHOL

See: Birth Defects and Alcohol; Underage Drinking

■ CHILDREN OF ALCOHOLICS

If you turned to this section first, you may be wondering if one of your parents (or another adult relative or caretaker) is an **alcoholic**. Here's a simple test; answer yes or no to the following statements:

- I often wish my dad or mom would cut down on or stop his or her drinking.
- I often feel angry about my dad's or mom's drinking.
- I often feel guilty about my dad's or mom's drinking, as if I were to blame.
- I am afraid or embarrassed to bring friends home because my dad or mom might be drunk.

If you answered yes to one of these questions, chances are that your mom, dad, or other adult caretaker has a drinking problem and may be an alcoholic. You are not alone. Nearly 11 million children and teenagers in the United States are growing up in alcoholic families, according to SAMHSA, the federal Substance Abuse and Mental Health Services Administration.

Alcoholism experts who study children of alcoholics—COAs for short—believe that they are at a higher risk than children of nonalcoholics (non-COAs) for having a variety of emotional and learning problems and for becoming alcoholics themselves.

COAs AND THE RISK OF EMOTIONAL PROBLEMS

COAs are at greater risk than non-COAs to suffer from depression, anxiety disorders, and psychiatric or developmental problems that require medication or hospitalization, such as attention deficit hyperactivity disorder (ADHD), a syndrome in some children characterized by inattention, impulsiveness, and hyperactivity, and oppositional defiant disorder (ODD), a related syndrome of socially disruptive behavioral problems.

COAs may also experience more intense feelings of anger, confusion, embarrassment, guilt, and isolation than do non-COAs. They may be more aggressive than other children, complain frequently about headaches and stomachaches, skip school, and engage in risk-taking behaviors.

COAs AND THE RISK OF LEARNING PROBLEMS

According to a 1997 report in *Alcohol Health and Research World*, some research studies believe that COAs and non-COAs differ most in the area of thinking and learning, called cognitive function by experts. Their research suggests that while most COAs fall within normal ranges on intelligence (IQ) tests, they may have lower scores on IQ arithmetic, reading, and verbal tests than non-COAs.

COAs also have lower scores on performance tests that measure abstract and conceptual thinking. In general, many COAs do not perform as well academically as do non-COAs, have lower grades, and are more likely to have behavior and adjustment problems in school, according to a 1999 article in the *Journal of Studies on Alcohol.*

COAs AND THE RISK OF ALCOHOLISM— GENETICS OR ENVIRONMENT?

COAs are considered the highest-risk group for becoming alcoholics (and drug abusers), and genetics (a person's inherited characteristics or features) is a big factor. Biological children of alcoholics who are adopted by nonalcoholics still have a two- to nine-fold greater risk of becoming alcoholics, despite not being raised in an alcoholic environment.

Compared to non-COAs, COAs have four times the risk of becoming alcoholics, according to SAMHSA. Sons of alcoholic fathers have an even greater risk for alcohol abuse, and they become alcoholics at an earlier age than their sisters.

Genetics, however, is only part of the problem. Environment also helps determine whether or not COAs go on to abuse alcohol themselves.

The alcoholic family environment is a chaotic and uncertain one at best. Poor parenting, marital and financial problems, poor relations between siblings, and the disruption of significant events, such as birthdays and holidays, can all combine to put enormous stress on COAs. Add to that the pressure of adolescence, school, friends, dating, and society in general. Is it any wonder that many children of alcoholics, with a lack of caring support, are especially vulnerable to drinking and alcohol abuse?

THE "ROLES" COAs PLAY IN THEIR FAMILIES

Early research about COAs focused on the unique personalities adopted as coping mechanisms by children living with alcoholism—especially those with siblings (brothers and sisters). Researchers identified four main roles that most COAs play in their families in response to the chaos and uncertainty alcoholism breeds. However, many of today's researchers believe these early COA labels are too broad and do not take into account the fact that every alcoholic family—and every COA—is unique.

Still, many self-help books continue to use these terms, which can be useful for looking at your own response to an alcoholic parent. Do you recognize any of these classic COA roles?

- The **hero or heroine,** usually the oldest child, who takes over many of the caretaking responsibilities of the alcoholic parent and who excels in school and sports;

- The **scapegoat,** often the second oldest child, who assumes the role of angry troublemaker to get the attention he or she feel deserving of and who is most likely to use alcohol and drugs at an early age;

- The **lost or quiet child,** usually a middle child, who tries never to cause any trouble, is often sad and withdrawn and has a tendency to be sickly; and

- The **mascot or clown,** frequently the youngest child in the family, who uses humor and clowning around to focus attention on himself or herself to try to diffuse the tension and anger in the family and who is most likely to need psychiatric help later in life.

Many COAs are not destined to be troubled teens or alcoholics. In fact, more than half of COAs studied by researchers lead normal, healthy, successful lives and never become alcohol dependent. The experts call this group resilient COAs, and they share many common characteristics.

THE RESILIENT COA

More than anything else, resilient COAs believe in self-help and know how to ask for help. They reach out to caring adults outside the family—for example, a relative, a friend's parent, a teacher, or a coach—with whom they can share their feelings and get support and advice. Resilient COAs are also good communicators, have a caring attitude toward others, and have a real desire to achieve. They make it a priority to get and stay active in school, sports, and the community. They seek out support groups where they can talk to other teens who share similar problems and ambitions.

Are you a resilient COA? If so, remember the first rule of survival: Resilient people know they cannot "do it" alone—they ask for help.

Q & A

Question: My father's been an alcoholic all my life. Does that mean I'll be an alcoholic too?

Answer: No, it doesn't, but you are right to be concerned. Children of alcoholics (COAs) are four times more likely than non-COAs to become addicted to alcohol if they decide to drink, and the sons of alcoholic fathers are at particular risk. Your best defense is to learn about alcoholism and the signs of addiction, look for help and support outside the family, and—most importantly—not drink!

IT'S NOT YOUR FAULT!

Many COAs believe that they are the cause of their parent's drinking, or that they can control or cure a parent's alcoholism if they behave a certain way—by getting better grades, for example, or by being a superstar on the soccer field or helping out more around the house. Sadly, many alcoholics often encourage this kind of thinking through their tendency to blame others, including their children, for their drinking problems. But children must remember that they are NOT to blame, and *no one* can "cure" alcoholism. Your parent has to want to stop drinking and has to ask for help. In the meantime, you have to take care of yourself.

The National Association for Children of Alcoholics (NACOA) suggests you start taking care of yourself by remembering the "Seven Cs":

- I didn't   CAUSE it.
- I can't   CURE it.
- I can't   CONTROL it.
- I can take better   CARE of myself
- by   COMMUNICATING my feelings,
- making healthy   CHOICES,
- and   CELEBRATING myself.

GETTING HELP

Information equals power! The following books and Web sites provide a range of information about alcoholism and growing up in an alcoholic family and offer suggestions for where to go to get help.

THE GOOD NEWS

Many children of alcoholics start life with a definite handicap. They may be justified in feeling angry or resentful at times. Fortunately, the clear majority of COAs overcome their disadvantages—and their resentments—and manage to build decent lives for themselves. They have broken the cycle, thereby freeing their own future children from the burden of an alcoholic family.

See also: Alcoholism, Causes of; Recovery and Treatment; Self-Help Programs

FURTHER READING

Alateen—Hope for Children of Alcoholics. New York: Al-Anon Family Group Headquarters, Inc., 1980.

Carol Carrick. *Banana Bear*. Morton Grove, IL: Albert Whitman and Company, 1995.

Edith Lynn Hornik-Beer. *For Teenagers with a Parent Who Abuses Alcohol/Drugs*. Lincoln, NE: iUniverse.com, Inc., 2001.

Richard Langsen and Nicole Rubel. *When Someone in the Family Drinks Too Much*. New York: Dial Books for Young Readers, 1996.

■ CHOICES, RESPONSIBLE

Decisions mindful of both positive and negative consequences. Some teens will decide not to drink at all. After all, millions of Americans manage to live normal lives with little or no alcohol. They abstain for reasons of health, religion, morality, or just personal preference.

However, teens who plan to drink can learn how to bypass the dangerous phase of alcohol abuse that other teens and young adults go through. If careful, they can learn how to drink safely *without* having to "learn from their mistakes"—some of which can be costly.

Alcohol has been a part of life since before the dawn of civilization. When abused, it has been a source of hostility and aggression, disease and early death, poverty and divorce, accidents and economic loss. But it has also helped millions overcome shyness and social inhibition; strengthen bonds with friends, relatives, and colleagues; or just relax and have a good time.

The majority of American adults, adding up the pluses and the minuses, have decided to drink. According to the 2001 National Household Survey on Drug Abuse, more than 60 percent of Americans between the ages of 21 and 29 had a drink in the previous month. Older age groups were a little less likely to imbibe, but not by much—53 percent of Americans aged 50–54 had a drink in the previous month, according to the same survey.

But buried in the mountain of statistics that the Household Survey gathers, one interesting fact stands out: While many young adults drink heavily, as people mature their heavy drinking and binge drinking decline.

Although only a small proportion of children 12–17 years old drank heavily, the numbers changed dramatically for the 18–25 age group, more than a third of whom were binge drinkers. Yet every age group older than 25 had smaller and smaller numbers of heavy and binge drinkers, even though the total number of alcohol users remained largely the same. By the time they were in their thirties, the solid majority of Americans who used alcohol had become moderate drinkers. They had learned to enjoy a limited amount of alcohol, without drinking enough to cause harm.

RESPONSIBLE DRINKING

A simple phrase has become popular in recent decades: "responsible drinking." It encompasses all the commonsense rules, detailed in this entry, that keep drinkers from harming themselves or others.

DID YOU KNOW?

Heavy Use of Alcohol Declines with Age

AGE	Any Alcohol Use		Binge Alcohol Use		Heavy Alcohol Use	
	2000	2001	2000	2001	2000	2001
12-17	16.4	17.3	10.4	10.6	2.6	2.5
18-25	56.8	58.8	37.8	38.7	12.8	13.6
26-29	59.2	61.4	33.3	34.2	8.9	9.2
30-34	57.6	58.8	28.0	27.2	6.6	6.8
35-39	56.0	58.7	25.0	25.7	6.2	6.1
40-44	53.9	54.4	21.9	21.5	5.4	6.0
45-49	50.8	55.2	18.6	19.1	4.8	5.4
50-54	50.8	53.1	18.4	17.0	4.9	4.2
55-59	45.8	45.8	15.8	14.3	4.8	3.4
60-64	43.2	45.6	11.3	11.6	1.6	2.9
65 or Older	32.0	33.0	6.1	5.8	1.5	1.4

Source: National Household Survey on Drug Abuse

There are two ways of approaching responsible drinking—as a goal, and as a means to get to that goal. Most people agree on the goal, but they may differ about how to reach it—especially on how to help teenagers reach it.

Nearly 30 years ago, the National Institute for Alcohol Abuse and Alcoholism (NIAAA), in a report to the U.S. Congress, came up with a series of guidelines designed to encourage responsible drinking behavior. It read as follows:

■ Alcohol is a drug that can cause positive and negative social, psychological, and physical effects.

■ The responsible use of alcohol can be socially, psychologically, and physically beneficial.

■ To drink or not to drink should be a personal decision. However, those who choose to drink have a responsibility not to damage themselves or society.

- People who drink need to respect the decision of those who do not drink.

- People who serve alcoholic beverages need to contribute to a healthy drinking environment and not "push" drinks on others.

- Intoxication is not responsible drinking. There is a direct link between responsible attitudes toward drinking and the alleviation of the problem of alcohol.

Almost everyone agrees with these principles. A lot of lives could be saved if Americans learned to take them to heart—and put them into practice. Yet principles need to be fleshed out with details: What should people learn to do, and not to do?

The oldest approach to alcohol education is to accentuate the negative. Most states have required alcohol education in the public schools for many years, often going back to the days of the **temperance movement**, when many Americans believed all drinking was immoral. For 14 years early in the 20th century (1919–33), all drinking was illegal too.

As a result, the traditional education curriculum has focused on the harm alcohol can do to the body and on the devastating effects of alcoholism on individuals and their families. Of course, teenagers do need to understand these facts. But they do not live in a vacuum. They know that most of their parents drink, and they can guess that many of their teachers drink too. They see alcohol served in most of the restaurants they patronize. Even if their parents abstain, they know through TV and movies that drinking is commonplace in America.

As a result, many educators now believe that the negative approach may not be the most effective with teenagers. Kids tend to shy away from lessons that sound like preaching—"Do as I say, not as I do" is a good way to turn off kids. Instead, some educators suggest, these teenagers should be clearly taught that drinking in moderation is an acceptable choice for adults, just as **abstinence** (not drinking at all) is an acceptable choice. They also should be taught what "drinking in moderation" really means.

David Hanson, a psychologist and alcohol educator at the State University of New York, is a strong advocate of teaching young people the rules of sensible drinking. He writes, "Teaching about responsible use does not require student consumption of alcohol, any more than teaching them world geography requires them to visit Nepal."

In that spirit, the following section describes the main rules of responsible alcohol use.

Know what you are drinking

Learn about the different alcohol contents of popular beverages. Wine sold in the United States has the percent alcohol listed on the label. Liquor labels show the "proof"; divide by two to get the percent. But be careful: Liquor bought outside the United States may list the percent; multiply the percent by two to get the proof. As a rule of thumb, a can or bottle of beer has the same amount of alcohol as a glass of wine or a shot of liquor. Act accordingly: If two shots of whiskey get you drunk, so do two beers.

You may not see the label if you are served by a waiter or a host. Be aware that a 12-ounce serving of ale typically has one-third more alcohol than the same amount of light beer; sherry has 50 percent more alcohol than the same amount of red wine; and bourbon may have 50 percent more alcohol by weight than most scotch whiskies.

If you are offered a premixed drink, find out what's inside. A cup of fruit punch may taste like a soft drink but may contain the alcohol equivalent of one or more shots of liquor. If you don't trust the judgment of the person who is pouring, pour your own drink—or drink something less "suspicious."

Pace yourself

Remember, your body can only process one standard-size drink in an hour. Sip your drink slowly. Dilute liquor with noncarbonated mixers, water, or ice. When your drink is getting low, add some more mixer or ice. If you feel drunk, stop drinking; or better yet, order a nonalcoholic beverage to help dilute the alcohol in your system. Always keep track of the number of drinks you've had—you can easily forget, when you are intoxicated.

Know your capacity

Women do not process alcohol as quickly as men. They can drink a lot less and still be "keeping up." The same is true for men or women who weigh less than average.

Choose the right time and place

Do not drink by yourself or when you are feeling tired, unwell, or unhappy. Try to drink only with people you like, in a pleasant atmosphere. Never drink on an empty stomach.

Don't drink for the wrong reasons
Don't ever drink to be polite, to be one of the crowd, or to show off.

Don't drink and drive
Or drink and operate heavy machinery.

ABSTINENCE

Millions of Americans are quiet abstainers. You would not know from the mass media, but a huge proportion of adult Americans never drinks alcohol at all. According to the 2001 National Household Survey, 80 million Americans did not have a single drink in the previous year.

For all practical purposes, people who almost never drink can be considered "abstainers." In fact, that's what the NIAAA calls anyone who never has more than 12 drinks in a single year.

People abstain for a variety of reasons. About two million recovering alcoholics choose not to have even one drink, for fear of risking a relapse into addiction. Some of their children also abstain, having seen firsthand the negative aspects of alcohol. Many other Americans have health conditions or take medications that make drinking alcohol dangerous or harmful. Others do not like the taste of alcohol, or enjoy the feeling of being even mildly "high."

Many more abstain out of principle. Some organic or health food fans consider any drugs, including caffeine and alcohol, to be contrary to their ideas of fitness and nutrition. Also, many athletes believe alcohol impairs their performance.

Some religious denominations either ban alcohol outright or frown on its use. These groups include some long-established American churches such as the Baptists, Mormons, and Pentecostalists, as well as communities of Muslims, Buddhists, and Hindus. The reasons they give for abstinence vary, but they share the goal of avoiding harm to their followers and society.

MAKE THE RIGHT CHOICE FOR YOU

The abuse of alcohol embitters the lives of millions of Americans. Yet even more millions have learned how to deal with this powerful substance by abstaining or drinking responsibly. You can learn too; a few intelligent choices today can save you years of trouble in the future.

See also: Binge Drinking Among Teenagers; Law and Drinking, The

FURTHER READING
Jane Claypool. *Alcohol and You.* New York: Grolier, 1997.
D.J. Cornett. *Seven Weeks to Safe Social Drinking: How to Effectively Moderate Your Alcohol Intake.* Secaucus, NJ: Carol Publishing Group, 1997.

■ DISEASES ASSOCIATED WITH ALCOHOL

See: Alcohol and Disease

■ DRINKING AND DRIVING

Being a new driver isn't easy. Driving comes with hundreds of rules and regulations. Experience is the best teacher, which takes a lot of time and practice.

Saying no to the social pressure to drink isn't always easy either. Some of your friends are beginning to drink—some of them may have been experimenting with alcohol since grade school or even middle school. They may have a couple of beers or wine coolers before a dance, during a party, or after a football game. They look and act as if they are having a great time and may not seem drunk. And they want you to join in.

Do you? Can you say no? If saying no were an easy choice, few teenagers would struggle with it. Yet they do. By the time 12-year-olds have reached the sixth grade, almost 50 percent of them have been pressured into having a drink. So what do you do, especially if you are driving? Stop a minute, think, and consider these powerful facts.

DRIVING UNDER THE INFLUENCE (DUI)

Drinking and driving, or driving under the influence (DUI), means that the driver operates a motor vehicle while *under the influence* of alcohol. Sometimes this condition is referred to as driving while intoxicated (DWI).

Every state sets a maximum BAC, or **blood alcohol concentration,** limit for drivers over which it is considered unsafe—and against the law—to drive. If you are stopped for suspected drinking and driving, your BAC will be assessed. If you exceed your state's legal limit, you can be arrested and charged with driving under the influence or driving while intoxicated.

The authorities take DUI and DWI very seriously. You (or your parents, if you are under 21) will have to pay a fine. Your driver's license will be suspended for a set amount of time or, in some cases, completely revoked. If you are under 21, you also may not be allowed to get a new driver's license until you reach that age. And you may have to do community service as well as attend a special driver's education program. Also, the cost of your insurance will increase greatly.

DID YOU KNOW?

Percentages of Alcohol-Involved Drivers by BAC Levels, Gender, and Age (United States, 1999)

Gender and Age	Blood Alcohol Levels							
	0.01–0.04	0.05–0.07	0.08–0.09	0.10–0.14	0.15–0.19	0.20–0.24	0.25–0.29	0.30+
Males				Percentages				
16–19	11.9	10.7	10.3	27.3	22.1	12.3	4.8	0.7
20–24	8.7	8.7	8.0	23.8	27.3	15.5	5.8	2.1
25–34	6.9	5.9	6.5	19.4	24.6	21.2	11.6	3.9
35–44	8.0	2.6	4.8	17.9	21.9	21.3	14.3	7.3
45+	12.5	7.2	5.4	15.0	19.9	20.1	10.8	9.1
Total	9.1	6.9	6.6	19.8	23.4	19.0	10.2	5.0
Females				Percentages				
16–19	23.7	10.8	4.3	20.9	16.6	15.1	5.8	2.9
20–24	11.6	9.6	5.0	25.1	21.6	17.6	6.5	3.0
25–34	10.6	5.9	3.6	19.7	27.4	17.9	10.4	4.5
35–44	6.3	5.8	6.1	17.2	23.8	21.3	11.9	7.6
45+	21.7	6.9	6.9	10.6	21.2	13.8	12.0	6.9
Total	12.6	7.0	5.1	18.5	23.5	17.9	10.1	5.4

Source: Trends in Alcohol-Related Fatal Traffic Crashes, 1977-99, National Institute on Alcohol Abuse and Alcoholism, Division of Biometry and Epidemiology, December 2001.

Knowing Your BACs—Blood alcohol concentrations

The National Traffic Highway Safety Administration maintains data on alcohol-related car accident deaths in its Fatality Analysis Reporting System (FARS).

The amount of alcohol in your system is determined by measuring your BAC, or blood alcohol concentration, usually with a device called a breathalyzer. This test shows the ratio of alcohol to blood in your system and is expressed as a percentage.

A BAC reading of .10 means that alcohol makes up one-tenth of 1 percent of your blood. Young drivers show measurable driving impairment with BACs as low as .03 and significant impairment with BACS just under .10.

Younger drivers are high-risk drivers

Younger drivers are twice as likely as adults to be in a fatal car crash. The younger you are, the greater your chances of being in a serious accident. According to the Department of Transportation's Fatality Analysis Reporting System, 16-year-old drivers have crash rates three times greater than 17-year-olds and five times higher than 18-year-olds. In fact, car crashes are the number-one cause of death among all young people between the ages of 15 and 20.

DID YOU KNOW?

Leading Causes of Death
for People Ages 15–20

Rank	Cause	Percent of Deaths
1	Motor Vehicle Crashes	35%
2	Homicide	19%
3	Suicide	13%
4	Other Injury	9%
5	Cancer	6%
6	Heart Disease	3%
	Total	100%

Source: Vital Statistics Mortality, Centers for Disease Control, 1997.

Many reasons account for these alarming statistics about teen drivers: inexperience on the road; inadequate driving skills; poor judgment and decision making; too much night-time and weekend driving (when the chances of a car crash are greater); and impulsive, risk-taking behaviors such as speeding and drinking and driving.

How drinking affects driving

Drinking goes to your head; in other words, it has a profound effect on your brain. Specifically, it affects a part of the brain called the frontal lobe, which helps you think clearly, assess situations calmly, and make rational judgments. The frontal lobe also keeps you from making really bad, impulsive decisions.

Your frontal lobe is your best friend when you are driving—but only if you do not add alcohol to the mix. Even one drink impacts how the frontal lobe functions, along with how well you think, feel, and react in a stressful situation. And driving, which involves so many quick decisions, can be extremely stressful.

Driving requires multitasking

If you play soccer, football, or basketball, you know what multitasking is. You have to control both the ball and your body while you are constantly moving. You have to keep tabs on your teammates and watch out for your opponents. You have to follow the rules of the game, plus keep your eye on the field, on the ball, and on the goal or net. Multitasking takes a clear head and a lot of practice.

Driving requires multitasking too. You need to visually track several different moving objects at the same time, you need good hand-eye coordination, and you need to perform multiple tasks—all while you maintain control of your car and obey the laws.

TEENS SPEAK

"It Was Only Lemonade . . . "

Jason and I didn't really think any harm could come from a simple celebration. We were at my house, enjoying the first weekend of summer vacation and celebrating that we were officially juniors. We each had two hard lemonades each (that's lemonade made with alcohol).

It didn't seem like I drank much at all. In fact, it was so sweet that I couldn't even taste the alcohol. Later, someone told me there's more alcohol in this hard lemonade—5.2 percent in a 12-ounce can—than there is in many beers.

Neither one of us looked drunk when I asked to borrow my dad's car. He gave me the keys with a warning to stay close to home. Instead, we headed for the Parkstone Skyway; it's a mile-long suspension bridge that connects our island with the mainland.

Halfway across the bridge, something totally unexpected happened. A front tire blew on the car. I totally panicked! I felt so fuzzy-headed, I guess because of the lemonade, that I couldn't remember anything I learned in Driver's Ed about controlling the car. I hit the brakes hard, and then the car went into a spin, smashed into another car, and hit the guardrail on the side of the bridge. The car stopped, but I was so scared. What if someone was hurt? Fortunately, no one was seriously hurt, but my dad's car was totaled. And I got grounded from driving for my entire junior year!

When you drink, those abilities are impaired. You tend to focus your eyes on one area only, and you lose most of your peripheral vision. Your hand-eye coordination slows down, and you cannot handle the wheel or clutch and stick shift as well as usual. Your reaction times are off, and you brake too quickly or too slowly. You find it difficult to pay attention to more than one thing at a time, such as reading road signs and traffic signals, staying in your lane, following the speed limit, and watching out for pedestrians. When a person drinks and drives, all the talents that make someone a good and safe driver, and a responsible adult, are diminished—or disappear completely.

How much alcohol is too much?

Most states have BAC limits of .08 percent. That is the equivalent of two or three drinks in an hour, depending on the drinker's weight and gender. Thin teenagers and females have a lower tolerance for alcohol. They can drink less than their friends but still have the same BAC.

By 2003, 19 states—with more joining the list every year—has lowered their BAC limits to .08 percent. That is two drinks or fewer in the first hour that someone may be drinking and one drink in each additional hour. These limits, of course, apply to *adult* drivers.

Fact Or Fiction?

"I never drink hard liquor like my parents do. I only drink beer. When I go to parties, I'll have just a couple of beers. I'm okay to drive, right?"

Fact: No, it's not all right to drive! One 12-ounce can of beer, one 5-ounce glass of wine, and $1^{1}/_{4}$ ounces of 80-proof hard liquor (the amount in a single drink) all have the *same* effect. Just one beer can affect how you drive. Your reaction time, judgment, and ability to think clearly are impaired. Two beers may put you over the legal BAC limit of .00–.02 percent for someone under the age of 21 and make you a candidate for either a serious accident or a DUI (driving under the influence) arrest.

Q & A

Question: I just got my intermediate license after having my permit and practicing my driving for six months—and I'm *still* not allowed to drive after 11:00 P.M., when the roads are practically empty! Why not?

Answer: Although the roads are less congested late at night, many of the drivers who are out there have been drinking far too much. How much? The rate of alcohol-involved fatal car crashes is more than three times greater at night (63 percent) than it is during daylight hours (19 percent). For all alcohol-involved crashes, the rate is five times higher at night than during the day. With those statistics (taken from a 2001 report of the National Highway Safety Bureau), you need a bit more time learning how to become a defensive driver before hitting the highway at night.

ZERO TOLERANCE LAWS EQUAL "ZERO" ALCOHOL

Experts have proven again and again that it takes much less alcohol to "influence" a teenager's driving. As a result, *all 50 states and the*

District of Columbia have zero tolerance laws for drivers under the age of 21. That means if you are in that age group, it is illegal for you to operate a motor vehicle with *any* measurable amount of alcohol in your system, regardless of your state's BAC law for drivers over 21.

In other words, if you have one beer over the course of an evening and then drive—and you are caught—you may face the same DUI penalties that an older driver would, even if he or she drank *several* drinks. That is another powerful incentive not to drink and drive.

The BAC limits assigned to young drivers under the zero tolerance law vary by state and range from a BAC limit of .02 (the equivalent of one drink or less in an hour) to a BAC of 0.0, which means *no alcohol at all.* The BAC of 0.0 adheres to the letter of the law, since people under the age of 21 are not supposed to be drinking at all!

Knowing the laws and penalties for DUI

Educate yourself about your state's BAC limits and DUI penalties for adult drivers. If you are cited for DUI, many of these same penalties may apply to you. They may be even tougher—depending on your circumstances—and can include vehicle impoundment (taking and holding a person's vehicle until a fine is paid), vehicle confiscation, (process of legally taking a vehicle), or vehicle forfeiture (taking away a person's ownership of a vehicle); special license plates or plate markings; and ignition interlock (a device installed in your car that measures the alcohol in your breath before you can start the car).

Some eye-opening facts

You may find these important facts about drinking from the 1999 National Household Survey on Drug Abuse useful; many of the facts might surprise you.

- By law, the minimum drinking age in *every state* is 21. But the number one cause of death among 15- to 19- year-olds are car crashes caused by drinking and driving.

- In 1997, 14 percent of drivers aged 16–20 years who were involved in fatal car crashes were legally drunk, with BAC levels of .08 or more, even though these drivers were not legally old enough to buy alcohol.

- Every 20 minutes, a person dies in an alcohol-related car crash.

- On any given weekend evening, between 10 P.M. and 3 A.M., 1 of every 10 drivers on the road is legally drunk.

- On weekend nights, any driver with a BAC level *less* than .15 (that's five drinks or less in two hours for a 120-pound male or four drinks or less in two hours for a 120-pound female) is *380 times more* likely to get into a fatal crash than is a nondrinker.

- In a typical year, more than 17,000 people are killed while driving under the influence of alcohol.

When fatalities among passengers and pedestrians are added to the annual DUI death count, the total number of deaths is more than 28,000. That's the size of many small towns in America, or the entire student population of a big university.

ROAD RAGE AND ALCOHOL USE

Road rage refers to a driver's overreaction to aggressive driving by another driver by retaliating with a violent act, usually an assault with a vehicle. This growing problem on the nation's roads is one that some people compare in its seriousness to drunk driving.

Alcohol, which intensifies feelings, is a major factor in many road rage incidents. Staying alcohol-free and following the rules of the road helps you avoid road rage incidents. Also remember to always wear your seat belt: It's the single greatest protection against road ragers and drunk drivers alike.

HELPING YOUNG DRIVERS
BECOME GOOD DRIVERS

Several years ago, traffic safety experts decided to address the problem of high-risk young drivers by introducing a driver education program that extended the learning process for teenage drivers. This program is called Graduated Driver Licensing (GDL). If your state does not have a GDL program now, it will certainly have one very soon. Thirty-four states plus the District of Columbia already have some type of GDL program in place.

While state GDL programs help new young drivers become skillful and responsible motorists, **Mothers Against Drunk Driving (MADD)** works tirelessly to keep young drivers safe and sober. Take a look at both programs now.

Major components of the GDL program

There are many steps on the way to getting your license.

Stage 1: Learner's Permit

- Be state's minimum age for a permit
- Pass vision and knowledge tests and complete basic driver's education training
- Travel with a licensed adult over the age of 21 at all times
- Limit your number of teenage passengers
- Observe zero alcohol law while driving
- Remain free of crashes and convictions for at least six months

Stage 2: Intermediate Provisional

- Complete Stage 1
- Be your state's minimum age for an intermediate license
- Pass road test and complete advanced driver's education training
- Observe night-time driving restrictions (for example, no driving after 11:00 P.M.; travel with a licensed adult during late-night hours)
- Limit your number of teenage passengers
- Observe zero alcohol law while driving
- Remain accident- and conviction-free for at least 12 months

Stage 3: Full Licensure

- Complete Stage 2
- Be state's minimum age for full licensure
- Observe zero-alcohol law while driving

Young drivers must demonstrate responsible driving at each level—each having specific requirements and restrictions—before moving on to the next one.

MOTHERS AGAINST DRUNK DRIVING (MADD)

In 1980, Candace Lightner's 13-year-old daughter, Cari, was killed by a drunk driver who had just been released from jail two days before for another drunk driving offense—and he was still carrying a valid California driver's license.

Angered by the injustice of the situation, and fueled by grief, Candace Lightner met with a few friends to discuss what they could do to stop drunk drivers. MADD was born, and the rest is history. More than 20 years later, more than 600 MADD chapters exist in all 50 states, as well as in Canada, Guam, and Puerto Rico.

MADD's advocacy and activism efforts have resulted in thousands of federal and state anti-drunk driving laws. Among MADD's most significant accomplishments are:

- Introducing the "designated driver" program
- Establishing a Victim Bill of Rights
- Increasing the legal drinking age to 21 in all states
- Instituting tougher DUI penalties, including license revocation
- Advocating for a maximum BAC limit of .08 nationwide
- Championing zero tolerance laws for underage drivers

MADD is unquestionably the greatest advocacy and educational organization promoting safe, sober driving. Its mission statement is simple and clear: "To stop drunk driving, support victims of this violent crime, and prevent underage drinking."

SAYING NO TO DRINKING AND DRIVING

Choosing to say no is a tough decision, and only you can make it. By taking over the driver's seat, you are accepting one of the biggest responsibilities of being an adult: You are responsible for the lives of your passengers, yourself, and the other drivers on the road. Consider the consequences, in the short-term and in the long run.

Is the trade-off for making a bad decision worth it? How much do you value your life, and the lives of other people in your car and in other cars on the road? If you are having trouble making the right decision, remember that help is available. Talk to a friend, a counselor, your coach, or a teacher you trust.

If you are ever stuck in a situation where you are the driver but you've been drinking or you have to ride with someone who has been drinking, don't hesitate to call an adult (even your parents!) for help. Although you may worry that your parents will be angry, they would rather have you call for help than put yourself in a risky situation. You do not have to go it alone.

See also: Choices, Responsible; Effects on the Body; Law and Drinking, The

FURTHER READING
Grosshandler, Janet. *Coping with Drinking and Driving*. New York: Rosen Publishing Group, 1997.

■ DRINKING AND DRUGS
Remember those old horror pictures on late-night TV, where a mad scientist pours two chemicals together into a flask? Suddenly the liquid changes color, bubbles up, and overflows the rim in an explosion of steam and smoke.

An increasing number of Americans are performing a similar experiment—by mixing alcohol and other powerful drugs in their own bodies. **Drug interactions** (the effects that each drug has on the other) can be very dangerous. Even worse, the results are often as unpredictable as science fiction. You cannot be sure what will happen each time you try another test, or repeat the same test one more time.

In real life, the experimenters often wind up in the hospital or in other healthcare facilities. In 1999, the Substance Abuse and Mental Health Services Administration (SAMHSA) reported that close to half of all patients who entered publicly supported alcohol treatment programs also had problems with illicit drugs (that is, drugs that are illegal, such as heroin, or medical drugs used for nonmedical purposes).

HOW WIDESPREAD IS THE PROBLEM?
Of the 320,000 Americans who began treatment for alcohol in 1999, SAMHSA said 62 percent also used marijuana, 26 percent used crack cocaine, 20 percent used powdered cocaine, and many more used methamphetamines (white crystals some people take as a stimulant), heroin, and a host of other drugs. Many others are still mixing away: Out of 12.9 million heavy drinkers in America aged 12 or older in 2001, 30.7 percent also used illicit drugs, according to the National Household Survey on Drug Abuse.

Treatment professionals have long noted the obvious similarities between alcohol **abuse** and drug addiction as individual behaviors. Eventually they coined the term *substance abuse* to cover all types of chemical misuse and dependence, whether that involves alcohol, illegal drugs, prescription drugs, natural or artificial chemicals, or any combination thereof.

Unfortunately, some teenagers too have fallen victim to multiple substance abuse behaviors. Over the years, as both alcohol and illicit drug use has become more widespread among young people, many of them have been combining the two.

In fact, most teenagers who consume heavy quantities of alcohol also use illicit drugs. The National Household Survey on Drug Abuse issued some startling numbers for the year 2000. Some 66 percent of 12- to 17-year-old heavy drinkers (meaning, they drank five or more alcoholic drinks on one occasion, on at least five different occasions that month) also used illicit drugs. More than 40 percent of binge drinkers (they drank five or more drinks on one occasion, less than five times that month) did the same.

Even some moderate drinkers who never binged used drugs, but not quite as many as heavier drinkers—about 20 percent. The only 12 to 17-year-olds who seemed to avoid drugs were those who abstained from alcohol as well. Only 4 percent of kids who did not drink at all (in the month prior to the survey) used illicit drugs. Fortunately for the health of American kids, that was still the solid majority of the population—83 percent of 12 to 17-year-olds, according to the Household Survey.

Statistics such as these can be very convincing. They show a connection between alcohol abuse and the use of illicit drugs. Does one behavior cause the other?

WHAT ARE THE LINKS?

The Household Survey figures seem to indicate that the more a teenager drinks, the more likely he or she is to use illicit drugs as well. Other surveys show that most kids who use illicit drugs experimented with alcohol first.

Stepping-stones and gateways

In the past, researchers believed that some drugs were "stepping-stones" to others. They believed that a person who drank alcohol would sometimes move on to other, usually illegal drugs and leave behind their drinking.

But more recent behavior patterns have led many of the experts to replace the stepping-stone comparison with another one: They call alcohol one of the **gateway drugs**, along with **nicotine** (the addictive chemical in tobacco) and marijuana.

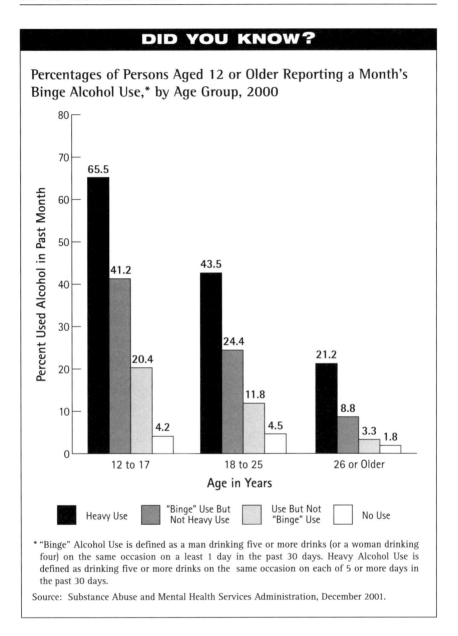

DID YOU KNOW?

Percentages of Persons Aged 12 or Older Reporting a Month's Binge Alcohol Use,* by Age Group, 2000

* "Binge" Alcohol Use is defined as a man drinking five or more drinks (or a woman drinking four) on the same occasion on a least 1 day in the past 30 days. Heavy Alcohol Use is defined as drinking five or more drinks on the same occasion on each of 5 or more days in the past 30 days.

Source: Substance Abuse and Mental Health Services Administration, December 2001.

These researchers do not claim that *everyone* who drinks tries drugs; many go no further, and may even stop drinking. But they have identified a path that most teenage drug users follow, starting with cigarettes and alcohol, then adding marijuana, and continuing to other common illicit drugs. For boys, the most common gateway is alcohol; for girls it is alcohol combined with cigarettes. Almost no teenagers use illicit drugs without first passing through these gateways.

Some experts in the field are uneasy with the term "gateway." First of all, they say, there is no evidence that alcohol use actually *causes* kids to try other drugs. It may be that the same reasons that cause some kids to abuse alcohol also lead them to use illicit drugs. The experts also fear that the public may forget that tobacco and alcohol alone harm far more people than illicit drugs, which most Americans still avoid.

Some of these researchers prefer the term **markers.** They say that alcohol and cigarettes are markers, or warning signs, that a teenager is at high risk for using other drugs as well. Using that terminology, the strongest marker of all is *early* drinking. Two-thirds of all those who start drinking before age 16 eventually use illicit drugs, while only one-fourth of those who wait until they are 17 to drink do so.

Reinforcement and cross-tolerance
Many kids who abuse alcohol may have emotional problems that make them likely candidates for drug abuse. Other kids may use drugs simply because they are available. But are there more specific links between the two behaviors? Are there ways in which alcohol directly influences a kid to use another drug?

One obvious factor is that anyone who drinks to the point of intoxication does not have the same good judgment he or she has while sober. If you were a young drug dealer trying to win a new customer, you could hardly find a more gullible candidate than a drunk. Even kids who know the facts about drug interactions, and who have no desire to pick up an expensive and troublesome habit, may put all those doubts aside while under the influence of alcohol.

Even if one drug does not actually lead a user to try another drug, once he or she does try it, the two behaviors often reinforce each other. For example, drinkers who have been introduced to marijuana may later use it in the hope that it may alleviate the miseries of a hangover. People who use **amphetamine**, a drug that can make their minds feel overactive or wired-up, may then drink alcohol just to calm down or fall asleep. Also, alcohol abusers may use amphetamines to wake themselves up after drinking too much. They are fooling themselves—they may feel awake, but their coordination remains unreliable and they should never attempt to drive in that state.

People who use more than one drug can develop **cross-tolerance** and **cross-addiction**. Heavy drinkers usually develop a **tolerance** to alcohol, needing to drink more to feel the same effect. Often, they become tolerant to other drugs too, even before they try them. Doctors often give higher doses of anesthetics (painkillers) to surgery patients who are alcoholic; a normal dose does not do the job. Alcohol abusers who "medicate themselves" with illicit drugs do the same— they need to take more of the drug to feel any effect.

In cross-addiction, people may use a substitute drug if their primary drug is not readily available. For example, heroin addicts frequently drink alcohol to relieve withdrawal symptoms when they cannot obtain any heroin.

Sadly, some doctors prescribe sedatives to certain patients troubled by anxiety and sleeplessness without knowing that the symptoms were caused by the early stages of alcoholism. Their patients often develop cross-addiction to alcohol *and* the sedative.

Researchers also suspect that a physical interaction between alcohol and certain drugs strengthens cross-addiction. Heavy drinkers who abuse heroin or barbiturates can sometimes slide into full **dependency** (alcoholism) in much less time than it takes someone who sticks to alcohol alone.

Alcohol and tobacco

The drug that seems to go "best" with alcohol is **nicotine**, the chemical that makes cigarettes so addictive. People who drink heavily almost always smoke cigarettes too. According to a 1998 report of the National Institute on Alcohol Abuse and Alcoholism, "Extensive research supports the popular observation that 'smokers drink and drinkers smoke.'"

According to the National Institute on Alcohol Abuse and Alcoholism in 1998, between 80 and 95 percent of **alcoholics** smoke, which is a rate three times higher than Americans in general. About 70 percent of alcoholics smoke more than a pack a day, compared with only 10 percent of the population as a whole.

Cigarettes are not illegal or illicit, at least for adults. However, they are one of the most addictive drugs on the market, as millions of people can tell you from bitter experience. And while the short-term risks of smoking are small compared with alcohol and illicit drugs (for example, you aren't as likely to have a car accident when smoking as you are when drinking), the long-term damage makes cigarettes one of the most harmful drugs of all. Smoking tobacco can cause lung and other cancers, emphysema, severe heart and circulation disease, blindness, and a host of other problems.

TEENS SPEAK

Which is Worse: Alcohol or Tobacco?

"People can sometimes be too smart for their own good," said Sorosh, a fourteen-year-old boy who lives in California. "Like, for example, my older sister."

Sorosh's family emigrated from Iran just after he was born. His parents honored the Muslim prohibition against alcohol and tried to get their children to do the same. "But ever since my sister started college, she hangs around with these kids who drink pitchers of beer every Friday and Saturday night," Sorosh said. "When my parents tried to argue with her, she just turned it around and talked about my father's smoking.

"She used to say that smoking was much worse than drinking. That's a big issue in my house, because my father smokes at least a pack a day, and we are always trying to get him to give it up. My sister would bring home booklets she got in school about the harmful effects of tobacco.

"As long as Dad smokes, she won't let him give her any advice. But in the end, the joke's on her: Since she's been drinking she started smoking too, just like all her friends who drink. They light up as soon as they get together and keep smoking all night.

"My sister still drinks beer on the weekends, but now she smokes every day too. My father has finally signed up for an antismoking program in order to get my sister to stop too.

"Now she listens to them a little more. Lately she's even skipped going out on a few Saturday nights."

EATING BEHAVIORS

Alcohol abuse is also often connected with another serious problem— eating disorders. Drinking can complicate and exacerbate **anorexia nervosa** and **bulimia**, which together affect several million Americans.

People with anorexia nervosa are unwilling or unable to eat the minimum amount of food necessary to stay alive and healthy. They usually suffer from the mistaken idea that their bodies are unattractively fat. Bulimia sufferers also are obsessed with their weight. They eat normally much of the time, but they are subject to cycles of binge eating followed by vomiting or other extreme measures to get rid of the excess food. The large majority of patients are women; often the problem first appears in the teenage years.

A large proportion of eating disorder patients, perhaps a third, are also alcoholics, and many abuse other substances as well. Researchers have not established a direct link between the two behaviors, according to a 2002 NIAAA report entitled "Eating Disorders and Alcohol Use Disorders."

HOW DRUGS INTERACT

In recent years, television dramas have given the public a new respect for the doctors and nurses who staff hospital emergency rooms. One of the most difficult tasks these overworked professionals face is diagnosis: Why has this man stopped breathing? Why does that woman have a dangerously rapid heartbeat?

Drug interactions are one of the most difficult diagnoses to call, mostly because they are so complicated. For example, low amounts of alcohol cause a very different reaction to many drugs than large amounts, while alcoholics (even if they have not had a drink that day) may react in yet another way. A person's age, weight, and sex can also play a part, as can the amount of food a person ate before or while he or she was using drugs.

Some drug combinations can have a reinforcing effect. Two depressants taken at the same time may make people so mellow that they pass out or even stop breathing.

Q & A

Question: What happens when people mix alcohol and ecstasy?

Answer: Ecstasy, or E, is a synthetic "club drug" that is somewhat similar to methamphetamine. Alcohol and ecstasy both dehydrate (remove water from) the body, and both can cause a rise in body temperature. When you add the two together, you may cause heat stroke and can damage your liver and kidney. If that isn't enough damage, people report that the combination makes for a severe "come down."

Other drug duos can cancel out each other, at least in terms of behavior: A depressant can bring a person down from a high so he or she appears almost normal. But beware: The same two drugs may reinforce each other internally, causing harm to the body. A few of the possible negative interactions with alcohol that doctors and ER staff have seen are

- Amphetamines: can cause severe gastrointestinal distress (stomach and intestinal problems); can lead to an alcohol overdose, since the amphetamine will prevent a drinker from passing out
- Barbiturates: can cause death from a reinforced effect on the heart or lungs
- Codeine: respiratory arrest (you stop breathing)
- Darvon: cardiac arrest (your heart stops working)
- Heroin (or any injected drug): high risk of liver damage
- Marijuana: greater effect on coordination and mental skills than either one by itself
- Tranquilizers: can lead to suicide or vehicle crashes, since coordination and common sense are at a low, even though the user may not *feel* all that drunk

Fact Or Fiction?

Inhalants aren't really so dangerous; other-
wise, they wouldn't be sold.

Fact: Inhalants *are* dangerous! Cars are dangerous when misused, and they're sold too. The fact is, various fluids, sprays, and gases that kids often use to get high can have serious effects. Whether kids use them repeatedly at one time, or frequently over time, they can lead to brain damage and even death—especially when combined with alcohol.

MOOD SWINGS

Therapists who treat mental disease estimate that two million Americans suffer from bipolar disorder, also called **manic-depressive disorder.** Even without touching a drug or medication, they swing between moods of mania, when they feel full of energy and confidence, and moods of deep depression or sadness. Often an incapacitating illness preventing the patient from performing the ordinary tasks of daily life, bipolar disorder is difficult for doctors to treat.

Ups and downs

People with bipolar disorder are in danger of becoming addicted to legal and illegal drugs. Even when not actually bipolar (and most people are not), they can still experience that kind of emotional roller-coaster if they abuse more than one drug. In many cases, alcohol and drug abusers can develop a pattern of behavior that is just as incapacitating, and just as difficult to treat.

Many drugs, including alcohol, barbiturates, and sedatives (such as Valium) are depressants. When their full effects kick in, people are less alert and may nod off. Other drugs are stimulants, such as cocaine, amphetamines, and Ritalin; under their influence, people feel wide awake and full of energy.

When people use illicit drugs, in a way they are "writing their own prescriptions." However, they can't usually control the dose very well. When they feel too manic, they may take a dose of alcohol to calm down or fall asleep. When they are too drowsy, they make take a dose of stimulant to keep them awake or to keep from feeling depressed. Before long, they are suffering the same effects as true bipolar patients. It can be difficult to climb out of this trap.

The mood swing of addiction

People can experience another kind of "mood swing" as they develop a dependency or addiction to one or more drugs. Therapists describe the four stages that teenagers go through as they experiment with a new drug:

1. Learning the mood swing. This is when teens first experience the mood change that comes with drug use. They may try to repeat that feeling through occasional drug use.

2. Seeking the mood swing. In this stage kids use the drug or drugs more to avoid negative feelings and stress than to experience the "good" mood.

3. Preoccupation with the mood swing. The need to change their mood becomes the main focus of the drug abusers' lives.

4. Using drugs to feel normal. The drug may lose its ability to make abusers feel better. It just holds off the bad feelings, which now include guilt and shame over being addicted, pressure to raise money to buy the drug or drugs, fear of being caught, and the painful symptoms of **withdrawal**.

COUNSELING, REHABILITATION, AND ABSTINENCE

In recent years the treatment community has become more skillful in diagnosing and treating people who abuse more than one drug. Counselors are trained to inquire about or seek evidence for cross-addiction, and most treatment programs and centers are set up to deal with the problem.

For the most part, therapists treat cross-addicted individuals the same way they treat those dependent on alcohol alone. Patients need to address the reasons for their harmful behaviors, and they need to develop healthier social and behavior patterns to keep them from reverting to drug abuse.

The main impact is on the medical aspect of treatment, including **detoxification** (cleansing the body of the effects of addiction) and any medicines used in treatment. People seeking treatment must be totally honest with therapists in order to allow them to devise the best and safest methods to treat each individual patient.

BAD COMBINATION

Both alcohol and illicit drugs can be difficult to handle and very dangerous. Combined, as they often are, they present a major challenge to physical and mental health that many people fail to overcome.

See also: Effects on the Body; Recovery and Treatment

FURTHER READING

Rosalyn Carson-DeWitt, et al. *Drugs, Alcohol, and Tobacco: Learning About Addictive Behavior.* New York: Macmillan Reference USA, 2003.

Judith S. Seixas and Geraldine Youcha. *Drugs, Alcohol, and Your Children: What Every Parent Needs to Know.* New York: Penguin, 1999.

■ DRIVING WHILE INTOXICATED

See: Drinking and Driving

■ DRINKING ON COLLEGE CAMPUSES

The college experience does seem to lend itself to drinking. On the average, high school kids who are planning to attend college drink *less* than their fellow students. But once they get there, their behavior changes. College students drink *more* alcohol than those in their age group who do not attend college.

Years ago, college was an elite experience. Only a small number of kids whose families had the means to send them could hope to attend. An even smaller number managed to obtain scholarships through hard work and luck. Today, the majority of kids in high school can expect to get some amount of higher education. Attending college has become part of the experience of growing up for the majority of American youth.

For the most part, college is a positive experience. Students gain the knowledge they need to succeed in the working world, and refine their social and intellectual skills so they can take full part in adult life.

For many students, one of these social achievements is learning how to drink sensibly. Unfortunately, some of their fellow students who drink fail that course. America's colleges are experiencing some serious problems with **alcohol abuse** among students.

If you are planning to attend college, try to familiarize yourself with these problems, so you are better prepared to handle them sensibly when the time comes.

WHAT ARE THE NUMBERS?

The Core Institute of Southern Illinois University reported in 1996 that 84 percent of college students said they had drunk alcohol within the past year, and 72 percent within the past 30 days. The legal age limit did not seem to matter. The numbers for the under-21 group were almost exactly the same: 82 and 69 percent, respectively. Among fraternity and sorority members of all age groups, the annual figure was 93 percent.

Many of the students were drinking substantial quantities as well. The same study said freshmen reported 5.7 drinks per week, but boys had 9 drinks compared to 4 for girls. Also, 45 percent of fresh-

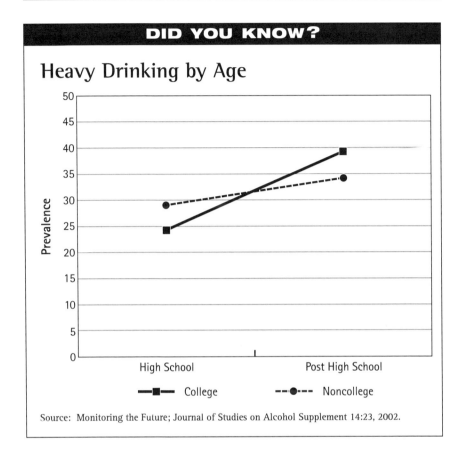

DID YOU KNOW?

Heavy Drinking by Age

Source: Monitoring the Future; Journal of Studies on Alcohol Supplement 14:23, 2002.

men admitted they had been involved in binge drinking (having more than five drinks at one time) at least one time in the previous two weeks.

The majority of college students manage to handle this culture without suffering any lasting damage to their physical or mental health. But not everyone is that fortunate. According to a 2002 report by the National Institute on Alcohol Abuse and Alcoholism (NIAAA), 31 percent of college students had abused alcohol during the past year, and 6 percent were alcohol dependent. As a result, each year

- 500,000 students between 18 and 24 years old were injured while under the influence
- 1,400 students in that age range died from auto crashes and other accidental injuries

- More than 600,000 students were assaulted by other students who have been drinking

- 70,000 students were victims of alcohol-related **date rape** or other sexual assault

- 25 percent of students experienced problems with their schoolwork as a result of drinking

- 150,000 students developed health problems

- 400,000 students had unprotected sex; a quarter of them were so intoxicated, they could not remember whether they had consented to sex

- Between 25 and 50 percent of colleges reported at least moderate property damage attributed to alcohol abuse

- Some 110,000 students were arrested for being drunk in public or from driving under the influence

CULTURAL ATTITUDES AND EXPERIMENTATION

For better or worse, alcohol is part of the traditional culture of most of America's colleges and universities. Long-established traditions of social drinking are passed down from older students to younger, through casual conversations, stories about the "good old days," dorm room parties, and socializing at off-campus bars and taverns.

These traditions were established in the days when most states allowed the sale of alcoholic beverages to 18-year-olds, exactly the age of most college freshmen. Going off to college and coming "of age" for drinking happened at the same time. The legal age has changed, but college life has not fully adjusted to the change in the laws. Needless to say, the many upperclassmen and graduate students who are 21 or over make it relatively easy for underage college kids to get access to alcoholic beverages.

New students find it difficult to resist these traditions, even if they are wary or skeptical. Most freshmen feel an exciting sense of freedom. Those whose parents had previously kept a close eye on their behavior now have to rely on their own sense of responsibility, which is not always up to the task.

College faculty members and administrators do not have the same role in monitoring student behavior as teachers and principals in public or private high school. Unlike the teachers whom freshmen may remember, college professors, lecturers, and teaching assistants feel no obligation to keep tabs on the on-campus behavior of their students, let alone their off-campus life. They are paid to teach particular skills or a specialized body of knowledge. They are not expected to help kids navigate the competing demands of college life.

Alcohol has always been part of the culture of fraternities and sororities. Drinking games, in which students (especially pledges trying to gain admission) drink dangerous quantities of alcohol in dangerously short periods of time, are notorious. At some fraternities in the past, no event was complete without a few beer kegs. Without empty bottles around, no one can keep track of how much anyone has drunk.

Fact Or Fiction?

The reason for heavy drinking in fraternities and sororities is that kids who like to drink are the ones who join in the first place.

Fact: The association isn't true. Recent studies have shown that once fraternity and sorority members graduate and move on to new environments, their drinking declines to a level that is normal for their age and background. Researchers now suspect that "Greeks" (fraternity members) drink more while at college because that's the prevailing "culture" among their peers and not because of any particular "fraternity personality type."

Of course, not every student pledges a sorority or fraternity. However, alcohol has always been associated with many other sectors of college society as well, from jocks to student intellectuals to the faculty. With the exception of a handful of institutions founded or run by religious denominations, few institutions in American life have been more accepting of alcohol than colleges.

Ironically, this acceptance can sometimes get in the way of the main purpose of these higher education institutions. Too much alcohol is linked to lower grades. The NIAAA reported in 2002 that several national studies conducted in the 1990s found that drinking was consistently associated with modest "academic impairment" (lower achievement).

In 1998, The NIAAA established a task force to investigate problems associated with college drinking and to recommend solutions. The task force concluded that the most important issue was the culture itself.

No lasting change was possible if colleges focused only on the individual drinker.

College culture may be changing, however, at least as far as tolerating underage drinking and abusive drinking at parties. Some college administrations have tried to limit advertising and other alcohol promotions on campus. Others have encouraged alcohol-free dormitories and social clubs. Several college towns have introduced tagging of beer kegs, in which sellers must keep track of purchasers.

According to a 1998 story in *U.S. News and World Report,* about 30 percent of all colleges had instituted more restrictive drinking policies in the previous two years. In one popular measure, colleges decided to fine underage students for drinking and to fine of-age students for having more than a certain amount of alcohol in their dorm rooms.

Fraternities are also feeling some pressure to change due to some highly publicized incidents of fatal alcohol poisoning caused by over-drinking. Expensive increases in insurance premiums, to cover alcohol-related lawsuits, may also convince local and national fraternity financial officers. In 1997, the National Interfraternity Council recommended that member fraternities set up alcohol-free chapters. By 2001, two-thirds of all national fraternities had at least one such chapter, and eleven were working toward a complete alcohol-free policy.

These measures are having an impact. The Core Institute at Southern Illinois University reported in the late 1990s that binge drinking had declined by 13 percent on campuses since 1980. Other studies have even shown an increase in the number of students abstaining from alcohol completely.

Some experts believe this news should be publicized more. In a web article in 2002, sociologist David J. Hanson of the State University of New York wrote that exaggerated reports of binge drinking are "dangerous because when young people go off to college falsely thinking that 'everybody' is drinking and bingeing, they are more likely to drink and to 'binge' in order to conform."

In fact, a 1996 study in the *Journal of American College Health* found that several colleges have had success in reducing problem drinking by simply publicizing the results of student surveys. Apparently, some students who discover that they have been drinking more than most other students find it easier to cut back. Some of them had previously believed that alcohol abuse was an *expected* part of college life. Conformity—doing what everyone else is doing—is sometimes hard to resist.

TEENS SPEAK

A Freshman Learns Fast

Sean, an 18-year-old college freshman, is living away from home for the first time. He still hangs out with a bunch of high school classmates who all picked the same state college campus.

"The first week of school, before regular classes started, we all went to a tavern just off campus to party. It was really crowded, so a couple of older guys didn't have too much trouble getting us in without getting carded. We weren't a big drinking crowd at Franklin, but somehow we felt that college was different. Like it was expected of us to get drunk. By midnight we were so boozed, we kind of staggered home.

"I had a roaring hangover the next day, but it was an exciting experience in a way. Like, now I'm one of the men. But then a couple of the guys started bringing six-packs into the dorm during the week, and we'd sit up drinking for hours. It was getting in the way of my studying, and frankly, I didn't enjoy it all that much.

"Then the college ran a student alcohol survey. I was averaging at least three beers a day, which I thought was more or less typical. But it turned out that only six percent of all undergraduates were drinking as much as me! I was trying to keep up, but with who?

"I was so happy to drop the mid-week drinking. I have more time to study, and to sleep, and even to get to know my new roommates. And I'm saving a few bucks too."

MONEY AND COLLEGE STUDENTS

College students as a rule have greater disposable income than their counterparts in high school. They are more likely to work (around 40 percent have jobs), and any money they receive from parents is likely to come in a larger sum.

In any case, inexpensive alcohol is readily available. Many off-campus bars provide low-cost promotions to attract students, including cheap or two-for-one beer nights. When allowed, they often advertise these specials on campus too.

The scholarly journal *Health and Place* reported on a 2003 study of eight campuses that measured the extent of heavy drinking (having five or more drinks on one occasion) against the density of alcohol outlets near the campus. As common sense suggests, there was a strong correlation between the density (number of outlets per square mile) and the amount of problem drinking.

For students at high-bar-density colleges, with competition driving down the price of a drink, heavy drinking may be the cheapest form of entertainment available. Two-for-one hours, cheap-beer Wednesdays, ladies' nights, and other promotions tend to perpetuate the culture of college drinking.

DRINKING AND RISKY SEX

Whatever you might think after watching TV shows about teenagers or hearing popular songs, many young people are not sexually experienced when they enter college. Almost 40 percent of 12th in the 2001 Youth Risk Behavior Survey (YRBS) had not had a single sexual partner (39 percent of boys and 40 percent of girls). Those who did engage in sex in high school generally had only one or two partners.

As teenagers become young adults, though, the situation changes. The respected *Morbidity and Mortality Weekly Report* of the Centers for Disease Control and Prevention reported in 1997 that 86 percent of college students had engaged in sexual intercourse at least once—and 68 percent within the three months before the survey.

These statistics sound bare and lifeless. After all, sexual feelings and behaviors involve so many complicated emotions—romantic love, the need for intimacy and affection, trust, fear, shame, and self-respect, to name just a few. Also, sexual behavior is influenced by powerful physical drives.

All in all, the factors that push people toward intimate relations with other people, or that hold them back, are often difficult to manage. As college students experiment with their newfound independence and freedom from supervision, some of them make errors of judgment. They may take chances they later regret, or find themselves engaging in activity they had meant to avoid.

Considering the risks involved, both physical and emotional, in being sexually active, doesn't it make sense to have a reasonably clear head when you decide when, where, and with whom to have sex?

Sexual behavior is considered risky if it puts either partner at risk of becoming infected with **HIV** (the **AIDS** virus) or any other STD (**sexually transmitted disease**), or if it can lead to an unwanted pregnancy. Examples of risky behavior are having sex with several different partners, having sex with a partner you don't know, having unprotected sex with a high-risk partner (such as someone who injects drugs with a needle), or having sex without using birth control. Every method of birth control carries its own level of risk; some can safely prevent pregnancy but do not protect against STDs. Without a condom, any sexual contact can be considered risky sex, outside of a monogamous marriage or similar relationship.

Risky sexual behavior is quite common on college campuses. The National College Health Risk Behavior Survey found in 1997 that only four out of ten college students always use a condom when having sex.

A 2002 article in the *Journal of Studies on Alcohol* analyzed the results of recent scholarly studies on alcohol and risky sexual behavior among college students. The authors found a strong connection between alcohol and risky sex, especially among those who are relatively new to drinking or sex—which is just the case with the majority of freshmen and sophomores.

The studies could not prove that alcohol is the *cause* of the risky sexual behavior. Other factors may include the individual's personality, the college culture, or particular situations that lead a student to drink and also engage in risky sex.

Even when other factors are taken into account, the article concluded that alcohol is indeed a major cause of "indiscriminate" behavior—the sudden, unplanned decision to have sex and the choice of unknown or high-risk partners. For example, "Young men who had multiple partners in the past month rose from 23 percent to 61 percent as the number of alcohol-related behaviors increased." For girls, the increase was even greater: from 8 to 48 percent.

The researchers attribute the connection to two main factors: the well-known fact that alcohol weakens one's sense of judgment, and the interesting fact that many people actually *expect* to behave badly when they get drunk. In other words, people sometimes drink in order to give themselves the excuse to behave in ways they know are wrong or dangerous.

ATHLETICS AND DRINKING

In the minds of many college students, alcohol and athletics go hand in hand. After all, liquor companies sponsor collegiate athletic events;

tailgate parties are notorious for consuming large amounts of beer; and college jocks have a reputation for drinking.

The notion may be a bit exaggerated, but not by much. According to the Core Institute of Southern Illinois University 1996 report, 88 percent of the athletes drink at least once a year, as compared with 82 percent of the general student population. But heavy drinking is more of a problem. According to college alcohol expert Henry Wechsler, more than half of male athletes, and close to half of the female athletes, engage in binge drinking.

In recent years, college athletic departments have instituted major antialcohol and antidrug programs. They are trying to break the connection, real or perceived, between sports and alcohol.

In 2001, the National Collegiate Athletic Association (NCAA) surveyed its member institutions about their alcohol policies and programs. More than 500 schools replied, and the results seemed encouraging. Sixty-six percent had instituted alcohol and drug education programs for athletes and 26 percent for staff. Nearly half had mandatory random drug and alcohol tests; athletes testing positive faced suspension or removal from their teams.

The same survey showed some improvement in the advertising situation as well. Eighty-two percent of the colleges reported that they did not allow alcohol ads on sports arena signs, and 77 percent kept them out of their game programs.

Q & A

Question: If college athletes drink more heavily than non-athletes, is that true for high school athletes too?

Answer: Not necessarily. In fact, an Indiana University study of 69,000 students in grades 7–12 in that state found that kids who participated in at least one team sport used alcohol at about the same rate as those who did not participate. However, the athletes were *less likely* to smoke cigarettes or use marijuana.

ALCOHOL AND SEXUAL VIOLENCE

Sexual violence takes place when one person forces another person to engage in sexual activity. Nearly all the victims are women.

Many types of sexual violence are no more common at colleges than anywhere else. But acquaintance rape and date rape have become a major concern in recent years on campuses across the United States. In the vast majority of rapes committed on college campuses (more than eight out of 10), the attacker is someone the victim knows—an acquaintance. In most cases, the crime occurs in a social setting, usually on a date.

A January 2001 Department of Justice report, *The Sexual Victimization of College Women,* reported that some 3 percent of college women are victims of rape or attempted rape each year. About 13 percent report being stalked.

Alcohol and, to a lesser extent, other drugs play a huge role in acquaintance rape. In the large majority of reported rape cases on college campuses, both those who commit the assault and their victims were drinking. Alcohol tends to cause aggressive behavior by an attacker and weakens a victim's defenses. With acquaintance rape, other aspects of alcohol come into play as well.

Most men know it's wrong to force their sexual attention on an unwilling partner. With some men, though, alcohol lowers their moral inhibitions; or they may excuse their behavior even while it is taking place by saying, "The drink made me do it." They also may associate alcohol with sex, feel more sexually aroused when drinking, and make the false assumption that any woman who drinks is always receptive to sexual advances. Sexual signals between men and women can be subtle and easy to misinterpret. If some men always think they are desired, they surely believe so under the influence.

When the woman is drinking, the risk of sexual assault increases. If a man and a woman drink the same quantity of alcohol, the woman is more likely to be intoxicated, due to differences in the way their bodies process alcohol. This puts a woman at a severe physical disadvantage if she tries to resist a sexual advance. It also weakens her decision-making ability, making her more likely to get into dangerous situations and less able to figure out how to escape.

As if alcohol isn't dangerous enough, drugs sometimes enter the picture as well. Some "club drugs," secretly dropped into a woman's drink, may make her unable to move or cause her to lose consciousness.

As colleges have become aware of this situation, most of them have begun serious education campaigns and have imposed more serious penalties on violators—a trend that is likely to continue.

Whatever policies college administrations may adopt, the practical responsibility rests with the individual. Female students must be aware of these risks before and during dates, even with guys they know. Male students should take a good look at their behavior, in advance and after the fact. They must learn not to use alcohol as an excuse for actions that may lead to suspension or expulsion from college, criminal prosecution, or jail. Also, they should face up to and reject any behavior that dishonors them and the values they uphold.

ALCOHOL AND CHUGGING: SUDDEN DEATH

Every now and then an isolated incident can break into national news coverage and spark a debate on issues that previously had been ignored. That happened in August 1997, after an incident at Louisiana State University in Baton Rouge.

A group of fraternity pledges went with their frat brothers to a nearby bar, where they drank a concoction of rum, whiskey, and liqueur. They eventually had to be carried out and driven home. When the campus police arrived at the frat house, they found more than 20 young men passed out. Four were taken to the hospital, where one of them, with an astonishing **blood alcohol level** (BAL) of .588, died of alcohol poisoning. Just one month later, a freshman at the Massachusetts Institute of Technology went into a coma at a fraternity party when his BAL reached .41. He died three days later.

Chugging, the practice of drinking alcohol faster than the body can handle, is believed to be relatively common at colleges. Chugging can take many forms. On college campuses, it is often associated with drinking games, involving swigging contests, spiked Jell-O cubes, and other ways of getting alcohol down the hatch as fast as possible. Often, some form of chugging is part of the **hazing** of pledges, which still takes place at some fraternities. In hazing, candidates for admission to a fraternity have to perform unpleasant, humiliating, and/or dangerous tasks as part of the initiation process.

Chugging is a potentially deadly practice. Even the most neutral and nonjudgmental experts, who may disagree about whether alcohol is a boon or a poison, offer the same warning about chugging— don't do it.

KIDS OR ADULTS?

College is the first phase of adult life for countless American teens, a time when they can make lifestyle choices independent of parental control. It is also a time when they must pay the full consequences of bad or uninformed decisions. If they are smart, they will come to college already prepared with information and sensible ideas to help them face the challenges of alcohol as mature young adults.

See also: Alcohol Abuse, The Risks of; Alcohol and Violence

FURTHER READING
Hank Nuwer. *Wrongs of Passage: Fraternities, Sororities, Hazing, and Binge Drinking.* Bloomington, IN: Indiana University Press, 1999.
Robert F. Salz, William DeJong. *Reducing Alcohol Problems on Campus: A Guide to Planning and Evaluation.* Washington, DC: National Institutes of Health, 2002.

■ DRUG ABUSE AND ALCOHOL
See: Drinking and Drugs; Drinking on College Campuses

■ EFFECTS OF ALCOHOL ON THE BODY
The body can handle modest amounts of alcohol, though the amount varies with age, gender, and size. It requires a delicate balance. Take in too much, too quickly, and a lot of systems go seriously out of whack.

Think of your body as a complex, almost miraculous machine. It can run like clockwork by itself, and even accomplish great feats–but only if you treat it with care.

METABOLISM
The process of **metabolism,** or breaking down what your body takes in, works like this: first, alcohol is absorbed into your bloodstream through the different parts of the digestive system–the mouth, stomach, and intestines. Then, your liver metabolizes the alcohol into products your body can handle better. Finally, some of these products get used or misused in the body while the others are eliminated as waste.

All along this path, alcohol interacts with the other foods and drugs it finds in your system. And it leaves its effects, visible and invisible, on the body.

Absorption
Each time you drink, the alcohol in the beverage starts to work almost instantly. Before you can even swallow, some of it gets absorbed into

the blood through the mucus membranes of the mouth. But 95 percent does manage to slither down to the stomach. The stomach, in turn, allows 25 percent to pass through its lining into the blood and pushes the rest into the intestine. That remaining 70 percent is gradually absorbed through the walls of the intestines.

A little bit of the alcohol evaporates out of the blood as it passes through the lungs. The lungs in turn exhale the alcohol into the air. Other tiny quantities evaporate through the skin.

When a person has one standard-sized drink on an empty stomach, with no other digestion work to do, the efficient gastro-intestinal tract (digestive system) can complete the absorption process in 30 minutes. But that is like running an assembly line so fast that the parts pile up dangerously in front of the next guy on the line—the liver. He just can't handle the volume.

A full stomach usually cuts the absorption rate in half so that the bloodstream has an hour to absorb the drink. Foods with high fat content are especially good at slowing down alcohol absorption.

On the other hand, the carbon dioxide in sparkling wine or some mixed drinks actually speeds up absorption, which is what gives champagne its reputation for making people drunk. Also, the higher the alcohol content of the beverage, the faster your blood alcohol level rises.

TEENS SPEAK

"I Just Had One Glass"

Heather won't soon forget the experiment in alcohol absorption which she "performed" last December. Her older sister, Sid, was taking her and her parents out for dinner but wanted to stop off first at her office's Christmas party.

Heather is 15, but she's a little shy in a room full of strangers, so she stood against the wall near the exit to wait for her parents to show up. Unfortunately, that was right near the punch bowl. "I just had one glass. It was delicious, like pop, and anyway Sid had told me it wasn't very alcoholic—two parts wine to one part fruit juice and one part seltzer water. We were expecting my parents any minute. But then ten minutes passed, and I started getting fidgety.

"I didn't want to eat anything from the buffet and spoil my appetite, so I took another glass of punch. After all, I've had two glasses of wine before, at Thanksgiving dinner, without any problem.

"But those two drinks one after the other, on an empty stomach, with all those bubbles, were a killer. It all went to my head in no time flat; I got so woozy I almost fell flat on my face. Sid and her boss had to walk me to the ladies' room to lie down. I felt so stupid, but I learned my lesson. I'm glad I was with nice people when it happened."

An individual's size matters too. If two individuals have the same type of drink, an individual weighing 200 pounds has a blood alcohol level that is half of someone who weighs 100 pounds. But the heavier guy retains the alcohol in his system longer, since his extra weight slows down the alcohol's elimination.

Men and women also absorb alcohol differently. Men have enzymes (active chemicals) in the stomach, which help break down alcohol before it can be absorbed. These enzymes are much less active in women. In addition, men's bodies tend to have a higher ratio of water to fatty tissue, so that the water in their body tissues dilutes some of the alcohol.

In other words, if a man and a woman of the same body weight have the same type of drink, the woman absorbs more alcohol into her bloodstream (30 percent more, by some estimates), and the alcohol she does absorb does not get diluted as much. Of course, the average woman is smaller than the average man, so the difference in BAC, or blood alcohol levels, is even greater, on the average, between men and women having the same type and amount of alcohol.

Differences in the reproductive systems of men and women also affect alcohol absorption. Women seem to absorb more alcohol into their blood during the premenstrual phase (just before a period). Women who take birth control pills also have higher levels of absorption.

One other important note for women: Alcohol has no trouble finding its way into breast milk. Any mother who is breast-feeding her newborn child should avoid alcohol.

Breakdown

Like everything you eat or drink, alcohol has to be metabolized, or broken down into chemicals the body can handle as nutrients or waste. This process takes place mostly in the liver, which removes as much alcohol from the bloodstream as it can at a time. Under normal circumstances, the liver takes about one hour to metabolize the alcohol in one standard-sized drink, whether beer, wine, or liquor.

If you drink more than one drink per hour, the liver does not absorb much of the excess. The alcohol keeps right on circulating through your brain and other organs, creating numerous effects on various parts of your body.

Heavy drinkers may develop some **tolerance** (the ability to handle larger amounts), as the liver becomes able to metabolize alcohol at a higher rate. But this strains the liver, which in turn can have other harmful effects.

EATING, DRINKING, AND CAFFEINE

Most of what people take into their bodies is classified as food—the fuel for the human machine. Normally, scientists consider alcoholic beverages to be drugs rather than foods.

Alcohol and nutrition

Alcohol does contain calories, however, which the body can use, while beer and wine provide traces (very small amounts) of nutrients. So what happens if you compare alcohol to food, for the sake of argument? How does it stack up? Not very well. You may have heard that red wine contains iron, but you'd need to drink about 30 glasses a day to get all the iron you need. And calcium? Fifty 12-ounce cans of beer give you all the calcium your bones could desire in a day.

The one food value that moderate drinking provides is calories—an average of 210 per drink. But today's teenagers get plenty of calories already. Also, alcohol instructs the liver to produce fat at a higher rate. Excess fat (from alcohol or any other source) winds up as deposits of unsightly **adipose tissue**, commonly known as flab. If your diet is already providing you with enough calories, you may put on a pound of fat by having 17 drinks over the course of one month.

On the other hand, heavy drinkers do not necessarily gain weight, even though half the calories they consume may come from alcohol. First of all, more of the energy from alcohol (compared with other calorie sources) gets burned up as heat rather than stored as fat.

DID YOU KNOW?

Harmful Effects of Alcohol on Nutrition

Too much alcohol:

- Causes pancreas to send fewer enzymes to stomach ➜
  Stomach fails to digest (break down) nutrients
- Damages stomach wall ➜
  Stomach fails to absorb enough nutrients
  Gastrointestinal bleeding ➜
    Loss of iron
  Stomach doesn't absorb enough vitamins ➜
    Thiamine deficiency can damage brain
    Folate vitamin deficiency alters lining of small intestine ➜
      Small intestine less able to absorb water, sodium, glucose
  - Impairs insulin secretion ➜
    Can cause low blood sugar in undernourished people
  - Prevents glucose formation from protein ➜
    Brain and other tissues starved of glucose
- Impairs digestion, synthesis, and processing of protein ➜
  Inadequate protein impairs cell structure
- Impairs fat absorption ➜
  Less absorption of calcium
  Less absorption of vitamins A, E, and D, which are normally
  absorbed along with fat ➜
    Vitamin A deficiency affects vision, and
    Vitamin D deficiency causes softening of bones
- Liver stores less vitamins
- Liver produces less protein, protein synthesis impaired ➜
  Cell structure damaged

Source: U.S. Department of Health and Human Services, 2000.

Moreover, alcohol can cause serious nutritional problems that work against weight gain. Unfortunately, alcoholics often neglect their diet too, making nutritional problems even worse.

Alcohol can slow down the absorption of some vital nutrients, such as vitamins A, B1, B12, C, D, E, and folic acid. As a result, these vitamins are eliminated as waste via the digestive system before the body can use them. Even moderate drinkers should be especially careful to eat a nutritious diet.

Alcohol also can affect the metabolism of protein, leading to the loss of muscle fiber. And if that isn't enough, it also reduces the breakdown of fats. To put it bluntly, heavy drinking often leads to malnutrition, although scientists are still not sure why alcohol has these effects.

Alcohol and coffee
When drinkers want to sober up, they often turn to one of the most widely used drugs in the world—caffeine. In other words, the caffeine in a strong cup of coffee is also a kind of drug, though much milder than alcohol.

Combining alcohol and caffeine may be a mistake. It is true that caffeine, whether in a cup of coffee or in certain over-the-counter painkillers, can stimulate the nervous system, including the brain. Taken in small doses when you are sober, it can make you feel more alert and energetic and can keep you awake.

Caffeine, however, has no power to reduce the level of alcohol in your bloodstream or your brain. Nor does it interact with alcohol in any way to reduce its effects. That cup of coffee may make you feel a bit more sober, but the alcohol is still working in the same way, and your reaction time is still below par. Mixing a **stimulant** (caffeine) and a **depressant** (alcohol) is a recipe for trouble. It may give you a false sense of security and mislead you into thinking you can drive safely.

Besides, too much caffeine can make anyone jittery and restless. When you combine the two drugs in your bloodstream, the results are unpredictable. One thing is sure: If you feel drunk enough to want to sober up, coffee simply does *not* make you capable of driving or reacting safely.

THE EFFECTS OF ALCOHOL AND MEDICATIONS
More than 2,800 prescription drugs are on the market in the United States and another 2,000 over-the-counter medications are available without a prescription. Many of these medicines should never be mixed with alcohol.

If the package label for any medicine—prescription or over-the-counter—says "not to be taken with alcohol," believe it. Alcohol can make that drug either useless or dangerous.

Bad interactions range from the mildly upsetting to the deadly. They generally fall into four types: those that enhance the intoxicating effects of alcohol; those that enhance the intended effects of the medication; those that inhibit or neutralize the intended effects of the medication; and alcohol-medication combinations that are toxic and potentially fatal. Here is a brief look at some of the more common or serious interactions.

Antibiotics are medications used to treat infections. Combined with alcohol, some may cause headaches, nausea, vomiting, and even convulsions. The effectiveness of others is reduced when combined with alcohol.

Antidepressant medications can help reduce antisocial behavior, anxiety, depression, eating disorders, insomnia, obsessive/compulsive disorders, and panic attacks. Doctors prescribe them for many adolescents and teens. This class of drug enhances the intoxicating effects of alcohol. At the same time, alcohol increases the sedating effects of most antidepressants, causing drowsiness, dizziness, and poor coordination.

Beer and red wine are in a special category when it comes to antidepressants. They contain a chemical called tyramine that dangerously interacts with a class of antidepressant drugs called MAOIs (monoamine oxidase inhibitors) to cause a potentially fatal increase in blood pressure.

Alcohol also increases the sedating effects of antihistamines, such as Benadryl, used to treat allergies; antipsychotics, such as Thorazine, used to treat delusions and convulsions; prescription pain relievers, such as codeine and Demerol; sedatives, such as Valium, used to treat anxiety; and hypnotics (sleeping pills), prescribed for sleep disorders.

Combining alcohol with certain heart medications and antiseizure drugs can significantly reduce the benefits of these prescribed medications and put people with heart disease and epilepsy, respectively, at serious risk.

Finally, the combination of alcohol and the most widely taken over-the-counter pain reliever—**acetaminophen** (sold under various brand names, including Tylenol)—can cause serious liver damage and even liver failure.

The bottom line when it comes to alcohol and medication is this: Avoid alcohol and always know what you are taking, why you are taking it, and what its possible side effects may be.

THINGS YOU CAN SEE

If you need to know whether someone has been drinking or has a drinking problem, you won't be able to tell by wondering about his or her metabolism or the activity of the stomach enzymes. But alcohol does have visible effects on the body that can serve to tip off friends or family members who care to be observant.

Effects on behavior

Subtle signs can let you know that people are under the influence of alcohol—even if they are not obviously intoxicated. Other symptoms may indicate a persistent drinking problem.

Many people can have one or two alcoholic drinks without losing their ability to perform routine, simple physical and mental tasks. But with each increased dose of alcohol, more complicated tasks become harder to carry out, even for people who don't act as if they are drunk or intoxicated. For example, any work requiring hand-eye coordination suffers—even something as simple as picking up a pen from the floor.

People under the influence of alcohol often have difficulty doing more than one thing at a time. They may talk clearly or walk without swaying, but they focus what attention they have on only one task at a time. They can be easily distracted and may have trouble remembering things. Their reaction times may suffer—which is what makes it so risky to drive "under the influence." And they may talk or behave in a manner that is inappropriate to the situation—for example, laughing, crying, or arguing over trivial details.

Of course, even when sober, some people are highly focused while others are more relaxed and easygoing. Some people have a steel-trap memory for detail, while others cheerfully admit, with a smile and a shrug, that they just cannot remember names. But it is the change from normal behavior that can be a sign of intoxication.

A drinker's eyes can be a giveaway too. Sometimes the signs are obvious. Alcohol can cause congestion of the blood vessels (too much blood) in the eye, so that the whites appear bloodshot and irritated. Or the eyes may appear overly moist and "glassy," or even unmoving and lifeless.

Some of the signs are less obvious, and may be difficult to catch at first glance. For example: When you are sober, your brain has an astonishing ability to focus and refocus your eye muscles as you move your head or as different objects come into view. Alcohol can slow down this complex mental function. A person who has had too much to drink often experiences blurred or double vision. When people struggle to see something within their normal range, too much alcohol may be the reason.

Even moderate drinking can have an affect on the eyes. For example, usually someone who looks to the side while holding his or her head still has no difficulty doing so. When someone who has been drinking tries it, the eyeballs often twitch or vibrate noticeably. Experiments have shown that the higher the level of blood alcohol, the less the eye has to move sideways in order to trigger this effect. Moderate drinkers may learn to compensate for these effects, for example, by turning their bodies toward you when you speak, rather than just their eyes.

Q & A

Question: Is it true that alcohol can shrink the brain?

Answer: Unfortunately, yes. Autopsies have long shown that people with chronic alcohol problems have smaller and lighter brains. CAT scans and MRIs of live patients show the same effects. When alcoholics who continue to drink are monitored over several years, their brains appear to get progressively smaller. The effect seems to be most severe in the outer layer of the frontal lobe, which controls higher intelligence.

Effects on the skin

Alcohol consumption can make some people's skin turn red. When the liver breaks down alcohol, one of the chemicals it produces along the way is **acetaldehyde**. This fairly toxic chemical is eventually broken down into acetic acid, which is harmless and can even be used to store energy. But as long as acetaldehyde is circulating through the bloodstream, it works its effects—increased heart rate, impaired judgment, and a redness or flushing in the face (caused by an increased flow, or "flush," of blood).

Some people have a reduced capacity to break down acetaldehyde. Even one drink turns their face visibly red; it also makes them feel ill. This trait is especially common in Chinese, Japanese, and Koreans, and among Asian Americans. But it happens to people of other backgrounds as well. Few such people ever become alcoholic—if a couple of drinks make you feel ill, you probably do not want to keep drinking.

Alcohol has still another unsightly affect on the skin—frequent bruises. They are not just the result of bumping into tables or door frames. Alcohol has a harmful effect on the body's ability to handle internal bleeding after an injury. Normally, sticky blood cells, called **platelets**, rush to the site of a wound and form miniscule clots, which keep the blood from leaking out of the artery into the surrounding tissue. Lab tests show that heavy drinkers have lower than normal levels of platelets. If the wound is near the surface of the body, blood seeps out under the skin, causing a visible red or black bruise.

A few people are even allergic to alcohol, or to some of the other ingredients in beer or wine. They may develop hives from only one drink.

More common than allergies is rosacea, a condition where the face becomes permanently red and pimply, especially on or around the nose. Alcohol is only one of many causes of this condition; but severe cases, where the nose becomes enlarged and bulbous (or bumpy), are often caused or aggravated by long-term heavy drinking.

Fact Or Fiction?

Alcohol warms up the body on a cold day.

Fact: The truth is just the opposite. After a few drinks, the blood vessels near the skin expand, giving you a flushed sensation, which feels warm against the cold. However, this means that your body is losing heat through the skin, heat that you really need internally. This is how drunk people can freeze to death from exposure.

SO MANY EFFECTS

Alcohol is a powerful drug that can dramatically affect a person's mood and behavior. No one should be surprised that it also produces a long list of physical changes to the drinker's body. Anyone who decides to drink should keep these effects in mind, and act sensibly to keep the risk of harm to a minimum.

See also: Alcohol Abuse, The Risks of; Alcohol and Disease

FURTHER READING

Karen Bellenir (ed.). *Substance Abuse Sourcebook*. Detroit, MI: Omnigraphics, 1996.
Raymond V. Haring. *Myths, Mysteries and Management of Alcohol*. Sacramento, CA: HealthSpan, 1995.
Lisa Wolff. *Issues in Alcohol*. San Diego, CA: Lucent, 1999.

▓ HANGOVER

A catchall term referring to the nasty physical symptoms people typically have the day after drinking a large quantity of alcohol. Once you have one, you will never forget how it feels. With any luck—and a little good sense—you will never suffer the health problems of an alcoholic. But unless you abstain from alcohol all your life, sooner or later you probably will have a hangover.

You don't need to be a heavy drinker to suffer from hangovers. In fact, light and moderate drinkers are the most likely to suffer, according to a report appearing in 2000 in the *Annals of Internal Medicine*. Inexperienced and first-time drinkers are also at risk, until they learn their "limit."

Hangovers are not only unpleasant to the drinker on the morning after. They can have serious effects on other people too. They cause more economic damage in the workplace—through absenteeism, lost wages, or poor job performance—than any other alcohol-related factor. Hangovers also are an important cause of neglect and child abuse by alcoholic parents: The hours spent laying in bed in misery cannot be devoted to caring for a child's physical and emotional needs.

SIGNS, SYMPTOMS, AND CAUSES

The most common symptoms of hangover are: mild to severe headache, nausea or stomach pain and vomiting, a dry mouth and thirst, muscle aches, physical and mental fatigue, dizziness, sensitivity to noise, light, and movement, sweating, tremors, and unpleasant emotions such as irritability, anxiety, and even depression.

If you experience all of these together, you may resolve then and there never to abuse alcohol again. More often, however, people experience only some of the symptoms, depending on the individual's personal body chemistry, the type and quantity of alcoholic beverage he or she drank, and perhaps the person's state of mind when drinking. As a general rule of thumb, though, the more alcohol you drink, the more likely you are to have a hangover.

A lot of different things go on in your body to cause so many different symptoms. One researcher sums it up as "dehydration; metabolic acidosis; hypoglycemia; disturbed prostaglandin synthesis; abnormal secretion of vasopressin, cortisol, aldosterone, renin, and testosterone; increased cardiac output; tachycardia; and vasodilatation." Translated into plain English, he means: The body has too little water, too much acid, not enough blood sugar, too much or too little of various powerful hormones, too much blood pumped out of the heart at too fast a rate, and dilation (widening) of the arteries. Quite a lot for just a few drinks!

Hangovers are considered a kind of alcohol **withdrawal**, the **syndrome** (set of symptoms) that alcoholics experience when they try to stop drinking or when they are unable to obtain another drink.

By the time the symptoms of a hangover are at their peak, very little **ethanol** (the chemical name for alcohol) or its direct breakdown product, **acetaldehyde**, is left in the body. But the alcohol has already done its "work" by causing dehydration, or the reduction in the body's water supply. Ethanol is a diuretic, a substance that gets the kidneys to drain water away from other organs. That draining causes the dryness and thirst, and probably contributes to the headache as well.

If alcohol itself is no longer in the body, what creates the other symptoms? **Congeners**, or impurities, are probably responsible for many of them. These organic chemicals are produced as a by-product of the manufacture of beer, wine, and distilled spirits (liquors). They stay in the barrel or bottle, helping to give each beverage its distinctive flavor. Some of the chief congeners are **histamines**, types of congeners found in alcoholic beverages that cause reactions in people who are allergic, and **methanol**, a congener that adds flavor to alcoholic beverages; another, found in red wine, is **tyramine**, a congener that can be dangerous for a drinker who also takes antidepressants and can cause headaches all by itself.

Some researchers now say that methanol is the chief culprit. Methanol is found in higher quantities in the types of beverages that usually cause the worst hangovers, such as champagne and inexpensive whiskeys. Furthermore, the time it takes the body to break down methanol into its toxic components—formaldehyde and formic acid—is about the same amount of time it takes for a hangover to kick in after you finish drinking. Finally, people whose bodies break down methanol faster seem to suffer the most.

Your hangover may be worse if you are tired or "overdo it" while you are drinking. As you drink, you become less sensitive to your own body. You probably don't pay attention to your body's signals that you need to stop partying and go to sleep. Even without alcohol, physical exhaustion can cause some of the same symptoms as a hangover.

Your general state of health and nutrition matters too. A healthy body is better equipped to handle a temporary "assault" such as too much alcohol.

Finally, your state of mind may have an effect. A study reported in the *Journal of Clinical Epidemiology* in 1993 confirmed the traditional belief that those who drink alcohol when they are angry, anxious, or depressed are more likely to suffer from hangovers.

Fact Or Fiction?

As long as you don't "mix drinks," you won't get a hangover.

Fact: There is no evidence that mixing different kinds or brands of alcoholic beverages has any effect on hangovers. You can get a nightmarish hangover even if you stick with one drink all night—provided you drink enough of it and the other factors are present. And if people only have a few drinks, properly diluted and spaced over a pleasant evening of food and sociability, they may well avoid any hangover even if, for example, they combined a predinner vodka cocktail, a small glass of draft beer at the table, and a splash of desert wine in the living room.

PREVENTION

To state the obvious, the best way to avoid a hangover is not to drink, or not to have more than one or two drinks at any one time. However, drinkers can take some other steps to reduce the likelihood and the severity of a hangover.

First of all, avoid drinks with high amounts of congeners. Champagne and inexpensive whiskeys have the highest, followed by tequila, brandy, bourbon, and red wine. Clear rum, better whiskeys, and white wine usually cause fewer or less severe hangovers, and gin, vodka, and beer (especially pale beers and light beers) cause even fewer. Gin and vodka are popular with many alcoholics, possibly for this reason.

Many theories have been advanced to try to explain these variations between beverages. Some of the theories even contradict one another. Here are a few: The longer a beverage ages, the more congeners form and the more likely the drinker will get a hangover; expensive liquors that are distilled several times are likely to be freer of the impurities that cause hangovers; prestigious "single malt" scotches cause worse hangovers than cheaper "blends."

The more experts you turn to, the more complicated the list becomes, perhaps too complicated. For most people, learning to drink responsibly—or not at all—will prevent more hangovers than all the research into congeners in the world.

People who drink hard liquor, such as whiskey, gin, bourbon, or vodka, should always dilute it with ice and a noncarbonated liquid such as water or juice (carbonation makes the stomach absorb alcohol faster). In addition, "topping off" a drink now and then with more mixer helps lessen the amount of alcohol one drinks overall. When it is diluted in the stomach, each dose of alcohol takes more time to enter the bloodstream. The mixers also help restore some of the water that alcohol drains from the body.

Drinking water is another popular preventive measure that seems to work for most people. Some advise drinkers to down a couple of glasses of water before going to sleep. Others say to drink one glass of water—larger than the wine or liquor glass—after each drink. Drinking water replaces some of the fluids drained away by alcohol, thus avoiding those symptoms caused by dehydration, possibly even headaches.

If a bad frame of mind contributes to hangovers, a person is better off drinking with friends or family in a pleasant environment rather than drinking alone at home or in a bar surrounded by cigarette smoke. That might be safer and healthier for other reasons (for one thing, your friends might keep you from driving); avoiding hangovers would just be an added bonus.

Experts do not agree on the value of painkillers or food supplements, such as vitamins, in preventing hangovers. Some experts warn against aspirin, the most popular choice, because it can irritate the stomach lining, which may already be inflamed by alcohol. Fizzy aspirin, such as Alka Seltzer, may offer a better alternative, since it spends less time in the stomach.

Acetaminophen (the medicine in Tylenol and similar products) may actually harm the liver if taken after having several alcoholic drinks. Acetaminophen by itself can be dangerous in large doses (higher than the number recommended on the label). When the liver is weakened by alcohol, even a few tablets can be toxic.

Some people swear by vitamins, amino acids, or herbs; others make money by packaging these common supplements in special "hangover prevention" form. Remember, unlike pharmaceutical (drug) companies, the makers of these products do not need to get government approval for their health claims. It is probably foolhardy to think that taking these products will allow you to ignore the practical steps of hangover prevention already discussed.

TREATMENT

A fully effective treatment for alcohol hangovers may never be found, according to one 1997 report in the *British Medical Journal*. The reason? The syndrome has too many different causes, and it affects too many different parts of the body.

Some doctors also fear that an effective next-day treatment would do more harm than good by masking the unhealthy effects of overdrinking. They believe unpleasant hangovers may help some drinkers understand the damage they are inflicting on their bodies. Such people may then learn to control or eliminate their bad drinking habits and avoid more serious, long-term damage.

However, some partial treatments may help. It often helps to drink lots of water the morning after, to restore your body's water balance. Sufferers can also try over-the-counter pain relievers other than acetaminophen (see the warnings in the "Prevention" section above).

When studied by scientists, some traditional remedies do not seem to work at all. Cups of steaming hot coffee, cold showers, or exercise do little or no good. But sugary tea, a time-honored folk remedy, may help counteract the effects of low blood sugar.

The most dangerous "cure" is perhaps the most famous one—"the hair of the dog that bit you." This cliché means that a person who wakes up with a horrible hangover should have a fresh alcoholic drink to deaden the pain.

There is a scientific explanation why this temporary "cure" might work. The alcohol in the "new" drink keeps the liver from breaking down the methanol from the old drink into the toxic chemicals that may cause hangover symptoms. Unfortunately, the new drink has its own supply of methanol and other congeners, and the whole unpleasant cycle begins again.

Bottom line: When you have a hangover, your body has just gone through the mill. All systems need to rest, at least for several hours. For severe hangovers, researchers recommend a good 72-hour break before taking a single drink.

In fact, starting the day with an "eye-opener," or morning drink, is one of the sure signs of a developing alcohol dependency. More than a few alcoholics finally understood that they had a problem when they felt themselves reaching for a bottle as soon as they woke up.

If the sensible treatments don't seem to help, get back into bed, if at all possible, and sleep it off. Time may not heal all wounds, as the saying goes, but it definitely does "cure" a hangover.

TAKE IT AS A WARNING

A hangover is neither funny nor trivial. The pain, misery, and disruption it brings can serve as a hint of the long-term dangers of alcohol. Smart people take the hint and learn to behave sensibly in the future.

See also: Alcohol Abuse, The Risks of

FURTHER READING

Raymond V. Haring. *Myths, Mysteries, and Management of Alcohol.* Sacramento, CA: HealthSpan Communications, 1995.
Gail Stewart. *Teen Alcoholics.* San Diego, CA: Lucent Books, 2000.

■ LAW AND DRINKING, THE

Alcohol laws have been around almost as long as alcohol itself. Even ancient civilizations regulated the sale and public consumption of alcohol, and so have most governments since. At the same time, the beverage has been an important source of government revenue through taxes or monopolies.

The United States is no exception to this rule. The first colonists who arrived from England brought with them a set of beliefs about alcohol and how to control its use. These beliefs have gone through many changes, and have generated years of passionate controversy.

In response, the laws have been repeatedly changed, at the federal, state, and local levels. And because the American population and public opinion are constantly changing, alcohol laws are likely to change again.

TEMPERANCE MOVEMENT

Though many of the English colonists who came to America were strict observers of religious law, they were not abstainers, or non-drinkers. The famous Puritan preacher Increase Mather wrote, "Drink is in itself a good creature of God, but the abuse of drink is from Satan." The colonists produced and consumed large quantities of beer, whiskey, gin, and rum. In fact, rum was probably the most valuable product manufactured in the colonies. Local governments encouraged the licensing and building of breweries, distilleries, and taverns.

After the United States became independent, the first major threat to its unity was the so-called Whiskey Rebellion of 1794. Thousands of farmers in western Pennsylvania refused to honor a new federal tax on liquor, which they felt threatened their freedom to produce and consume as much whiskey as they chose.

By the early 1800s, Americans were drinking about three times as much liquor, beer, and wine as they do today, and alcohol abuse was commonplace. In reaction, a **temperance movement** began to emerge, especially among churchgoers. The movement condemned alcohol abuse as a source of disease and poverty. As alternatives, it promoted temperance, or moderation, in drinking, and encouraged the use of nonalcoholic beverages such as root beer.

It was an era of reformist movements, such as abolitionism (which opposed slavery), prison reform, and women's rights. Many women were active in the temperance movement, which spread throughout United States and to many European countries.

By the middle of the 1800s, the movement began to advocate **prohibition**—a complete ban on the sale or drinking of alcohol. Maine became the first state to outlaw alcohol, in 1851, and several other states followed.

The founding of the Prohibition Party in 1869 and the Women's Christian Temperance Union in 1874 signaled the start of a major political campaign. For the next 60 years, alcohol remained one of the most important issues on the political agenda, affecting every presidential election for decades. The issues split the country into regional, religious, and urban or rural factions.

In the early 1900s, the movement gained support from social reformers who wanted to protect the working classes from alcoholism, political reformers who saw alcohol and taverns as a key part of corrupt political machines, and business owners looking to reduce absenteeism and injuries in their factories.

VOLSTEAD ACT OF 1919

During World War I (1917–1918), the government declared wartime prohibition, in part to divert grain from alcohol production to food. Then, in 1919, the Eighteenth Amendment to the U.S. Constitution was ratified, outlawing the "manufacture, sale and transportation of intoxicating liquors." Later that year Congress passed the famous Volstead Act, which put the amendment into effect. What people called "the great experiment" of Prohibition was under way.

The Volstead Act defined "intoxicating liquors" as any beverage whose alcohol content was 0.5 percent or more, which made beer and wine, as well as hard liquor, illegal. But the Eighteenth Amendment did not make it illegal to possess liquor for personal use, and the Volstead Act did not generally allow searches of individual homes. As a result, many people began to make their own alcoholic beverages. Businesses could legally produce alcohol for industrial and scientific purposes and for sacramental use, for example by Catholic priests or Jewish rabbis. Doctors also could prescribe wine or liquor for "medicinal" reasons. All these loopholes eventually allowed large quantities of legally manufactured alcohol to be sidetracked for sale by bootleggers, the importers and bulk sellers of illegal alcohol, and speakeasies, or illegal saloons.

The federal government set up a Prohibition Bureau in the Treasury Department to enforce the Volstead Act. Some 170,000 saloons were shut down across the country. Contrary to popular belief, Prohibition was successfully enforced in much of the country, and it achieved many of its aims. Arrests for public drunkenness declined dramatically. Hospital admissions for alcoholism, alcohol psychosis (an episode of severe mental illness), and alcohol-related diseases fell by more than half within a few years.

Prohibitionists claimed that there were fewer broken homes caused by lost wages and domestic violence. The evidence shows that alcohol consumption fell the most among poorer people, who could not afford the high price of illegal alcohol. Even after Prohibition was repealed by the Twenty-first Amendment, and sales resumed in 1934, consumption did not immediately rise to pre-1919 levels, which suggests that many people had lost the habit of drinking.

The tales of Prohibition crime made popular in many gangster movies have been somewhat exaggerated, according to some historians. Organized criminal mobs ran illegal rackets in the big cities long before Prohibition, and murder rates had already risen well before 1919.

But the law did make millions of ordinary citizens partners in crime. Many immigrant ethnic groups refused to give up their cultural attachment to wine, beer, or whiskey. These drinks also remained an essential part of social life for middle-class people in the cities. Without regulation by the government, much of the alcohol sold was of poor quality, and some was even dangerously toxic.

Fact Or Fiction?

During the 1920s, when Prohibition was in effect in the United States, people drank more than they ever had before.

Fact: Actually, this is not true. Evidence suggests that there was a sizable reduction in drinking during Prohibition. In many states, alcoholic beverages were not easy to obtain. In all regions, prices went up, and poorer people simply could not afford to drink.

These factors, plus the publicity over Prohibition-related crime and violence, began to make the policy unpopular. When the Great Depression began in 1929, closing factories and throwing millions of people out of work, Prohibition became an economic issue. Opponents held out the hope that repeal would mean new jobs and tax revenues. In 1933, the Twenty-first Amendment to the Constitution was approved, repealing the Eighteenth (Prohibition) Amendment.

Some states continued Prohibition on a statewide or local level; Mississippi was the last state to repeal, in 1966. Most states adopted new laws to limit the sale of alcohol. They restricted the hours and days that taverns could operate, or required taverns to serve food. Some states even banned any sales outside of state-owned "package stores," which never sold by the drink. Many of these laws remain in effect today.

PUBLIC INTOXICATION:
CRIMINAL OR VICTIM?

After the repeal of Prohibition, state and local governments continued to deal with alcohol abuse, but their focus shifted. Public intoxication and its dangerous effects once again became the main alcohol-related issue in law and government.

Public drunkenness laws go back more than 300 years, to the first public intoxication statute in England in 1606. In one form or another, these laws always remained on the books, in the United States as well. By the early 1960s, police officers in every state were arresting a total of two million people a year for the crime of public intoxication.

However, public opinion had begun to change, partly due to the effort of such groups as A.A., or **Alcoholics Anonymous**. Most people now came to believe that alcoholism should be treated as a disease. They wanted intoxicated people, especially homeless derelicts, to be treated with compassion. They wanted to offer them treatment rather than simply arresting them and allowing them to "dry out" (become sober) in a jail cell.

Despite this public change, the U.S. Supreme Court in 1968 narrowly supported arrests for drunkenness. Partly in response, Congress passed the Alcoholic Rehabilitation Act of 1968. This law was followed two years later by a more comprehensive law that called for major new efforts in research and treatment, and set up the National Institute on Alcohol Abuse and Alcoholism (NIAAA).

Still another 1970s federal law, the Uniform Alcoholism and Intoxication Act, encouraged states to change their approach as well. The majority of states eventually fell in line, removing simple intoxication from the list of crimes, and setting up **detoxification** and rehabilitation programs.

In practice, many public drunks refuse voluntary treatment, and police officers frequently arrest them on "public nuisance" charges. In any case, alcohol researchers have not yet found new, more effective treatment methods for putting a complete stop to alcohol abuse.

In the 1980s, private citizens whose families had suffered from **fetal alcohol syndrome** and other drinking-related diseases began suing manufacturers and sellers. In response, Congress passed a law requiring health warnings on all alcohol containers.

In recent years, dramatic and effective campaigns by groups such as **Mothers Against Drunk Driving (MADD)** convinced states to raise the minimum drinking age to 21. At the same time, local and state police have worked with judges and juries to strictly enforce drunken driving laws. Following these changes, the rate of fatal alcohol-related car crashes sharply declined.

ZERO TOLERANCE

During the 1980s, the federal government launched a "war on drugs," designed to eliminate the distribution and sale of illegal drugs. It was a response to the alarming increase in drug abuse and addiction, especially among young people.

In that climate, "**zero tolerance**" became a popular slogan among the public: People wanted the government, school systems, and employers to crack down on *any* violation of the drug laws. For example, they wanted students to be punished, even suspended from school, if they were found with any amount of drugs on school property. Employers began introducing drug tests for new or current employees. Any trace of drugs in urine would be grounds for dismissal.

Over time, the idea spread to other areas of concern, including alcohol. Many states now have zero tolerance for under-21 drivers—they can be prosecuted for having even the smallest non-zero **BAL**, or **blood alcohol level**, while driving. Under pressure from parents concerned about a safe, healthy environment for their children, many school systems have issued zero-tolerance policies against alcohol, illegal drugs, violence, and guns.

Q & A

Question: What is the legal drinking age in Canada?

Answer: Each province in Canada regulates alcohol as it sees fit. Three provinces allow drinking at 18: Quebec, Manitoba, and Alberta. All the rest have a legal age of 19. Up until 1970, most provinces maintained a legal minimum of 20 or 21; nine of the 10 provinces lowered the minimum in the early 1970s.

However, some parents, supported by political activists, criticize zero tolerance. They want the government to concentrate on prosecuting the major sellers of illegal drugs rather than the individual users, and they want the schools to focus on alcohol abuses, such as drunkenness or sales on school property.

These opponents have publicized cases of over-eager enforcement, such as the student who was suspended for using mouthwash in the locker room because it contained alcohol (as most popular brands do). Such cases, they say, are evidence of a "prohibition" mentality.

The schools are caught in the middle. Zero-tolerance policies can sometimes be unfair, but they also protect schools against liability (legal responsibility). For example, if a school is sued when a student who drinks on school property is injured, the administration must show that it made every effort to prevent such events from taking place. The controversy continues to spark heated debate.

A BALANCING ACT

Over the centuries, the American legal system has had to adjust to changing currents of public opinion about alcohol. From broad acceptance to prohibition, from a policy of arrest to one of treatment, and now to zero tolerance for young drinkers, the laws have been continually refined. While people still debate the means, most citizens today agree on the goal: to balance the desires of individual to drink against the general interest in health, safety, and public order.

See also: Alcohol and Disease; Drinking and Driving; Self-Help Programs

FURTHER READING

Andrew Barr. *Drink: A Social History of America*. New York: Carroll and Graf, 1999.

R. Barri Flowers. *Drugs, Alcohol and Criminality in American Society*. Jefferson, NC: McFarland, 1999.

▓ LEGAL ISSUES
See: Law and Drinking, The

▓ MEDIA, THE AND ALCOHOL
See: Advertising and Counteradvertising Campaigns

■ PEER PRESSURE AND ALCOHOL

The experience a person has of feeling forced, or compelled, to act the same as the social group to which he or she belongs is known as peer pressure. Face it—everyone likes to belong. Human beings are "social animals," according to scientists. People huddle together for comfort, safety, and because they enjoy one another's company. No one wants to feel left out or excluded from family, class, team, or coworkers.

As social animals, teenagers may be the most "human" of all age groups. They love to hang out with friends, to share good times, to help one another over the rough spots, and to compare notes about all the new things they are finding out about life. There aren't many skills that a teen can learn that are more important than finding and keeping good friends. They deserve your loyalty, and they owe you loyalty in return.

However, people aren't *just* social animals. They are individuals too. An important skill that people need to learn as teens is finding the right balance between belonging to a group and making one's own decisions as an individual. A teen needs to be his or her own person within the family, and among friends too.

LISTENING TO OTHERS

When you were a kid, you probably thought your parents knew everything there was to know. Then, after you spent a few years in school, you realized that they didn't always have all the answers, however much they loved you and however much you respected them. The world had changed a little since they were your age; in some areas, your teachers were the experts now.

Now that you have reached your teens, your life is more complicated. Your parents still have their opinions. Your teachers have their own points of view—and you usually have a new set of teachers every year. You watch television, listen to the radio, and see movies, and you read books, newspapers, and magazines. In addition to all these other sources of information, you have your friends, who are part of your peer group, people your own age in your community.

Your peers are the unchallenged experts in lots of subjects. They usually can tell you the best music to listen to. They know what clothing looks good on you and what looks hopelessly nerdy. They may have a good idea about who the best teachers are in your school, or what part-time jobs are available in your neighborhood. They can even help you navigate through dating, romance, and sex, and keep you from making embarrassing mistakes.

Very often, though, your peers will influence you by their words or by their example, even on subjects where they may not have so much knowledge—for example, alcohol or illegal drugs. There's no reason to *ignore* their opinions, whether on the risks of alcohol or its possible benefits. But they probably do not have the whole picture.

Some of your friends may in fact know some pieces of the puzzle better than your parents or teachers. They may be more familiar with the names and types of the latest "designer" or "club drugs," and where to get them. Your peers may know where underage kids can get alcoholic beverages, and where they can drink with less chance of getting caught. If your parents don't drink much, or don't drink at all, you may have friends that are more knowledgeable about the different types and brands of alcoholic beverages.

Just as your parents "don't know everything," however, your friends can be wrong too. Especially when it comes to long-term issues such as substance **abuse**.

Teens' knowledge about substance abuse is short-term. It may take several years for alcohol to cause serious physical harm and therefore cannot be something that teenagers know from their own personal experience. Nor do they always understand the damage it can do to family and work life.

And even if you assume, for argument's sake, that your friends know what's best for them, they may not know what's best for you.

You are a unique person, with your own needs, values, and goals. You have your own body, which may react differently to alcohol. You may have a family history of alcohol abuse, or you may have a family tradition of abstention (no alcohol); in either case, you may have good reasons to abstain, for now. Doing well on tomorrow's midterm exam may be a higher priority for you than for some of your friends; or maybe they are so smart they can ace the test even with a hangover. Are you sure *you* can?

MANIPULATION BY PEERS

When friends talk, they should honestly say what is on their minds. Sometimes, however, even friends can have hidden agendas. In other words, they may try to manipulate you—make you do something you really did not want to do by telling you lies or only part of the truth.

Kids who drink or use illegal drugs may have several different reasons for manipulating you into joining them. They may feel they have protection in numbers: You might not tell on them if you're involved too. They may feel unsure that what they are doing is really safe, smart, or all that much fun; if they can convince you to join them, it may relieve their own doubts. And finally, misery loves company. Kids who are starting to feel the negative, harmful effects of alcohol abuse may not want to face them alone. Getting you into the same mess is not the best way to deal with their problem, but it may seem like a good idea to them.

Anyone who tries to manipulate you into doing something against your better judgment usually tries to play on your fears and emotional needs, including:

The fear of losing friends. You may be afraid of losing the friend who is manipulating you, or other friends, if you don't go along with his or her behavior.

The need to be popular, to be part of a crowd. You may not really want to drink, or to drink too much, but you may be willing to, if you think that's the price you have to pay to join a group. (But think of this: According to Minnesota prevention specialist Kris Van Hoof, "The easiest group to belong to is the users. They accept pretty much anybody. As long as you drink or use, you're in." Is that the group you *want* to belong to?)

The fear of looking like a geek. You may want to turn down alcohol simply because it doesn't make sense for you now. But if you don't drink, will people think you're a nerd? Don't wind up *doing* something stupid just to avoid *looking* stupid.

The fear of being different. If you think *everyone* does it, you may not have the strength to abstain.

The need to be polite. No one likes to hurt or insult their friends by turning down their offer of a drink. No one wants to seem "holier than thou."

The need for love and attention from the opposite sex. A friend may tell you that drinking makes you less shy, improves your sexual performance, or makes you more attractive. Even if you think that sounds off-base, you might *want* to believe it enough to try. If your friend really wants to manipulate you, he or she may offer you a drink in front of someone he or she knows you like. That is very tough to resist if the other person is drinking too.

It is also hard to resist when you happen to be feeling low, depressed, or anxious. You may be especially open to manipulation at times like those.

Q & A

Question: How can I turn down a drink from my best friend?

Answer: The easy answer is, you should be comfortable about being honest with a good friend: just say what you feel. But sometimes your friend might be insulted or annoyed anyway. If your values, not to say your health and safety, are important to you, you may just have to take that chance. If you have to face the same question over and over, maybe it's time for a serious talk—or time to seek out new friends.

RESISTING PEER PRESSURE

It is hard to say no to someone you like, but you may as well learn that skill while you are young. What words should you use? Whatever feels comfortable for you. Here are some lines that other kids have come up with. They won't all work every time, but they may inspire you to invent some lines of your own. Think it over *before* you get into a situation, so you are prepared when the time comes.

- Don't turn down your friend, just turn down the alcohol. For example, you might say, "I like hanging with you, but I just don't like getting drunk," or "We're friends, but we don't have to do everything together."

- Offer to do something else. "Let's go eat; let's go to a movie; let's call so-and-so." If your friends say no, tell them they can join up with you later.

- Give a good excuse. "I can't"; "I have to study tonight"; "I'm taking prescription drugs and I can't drink"; or "I'm in training" are always handy (provided they're true).

- Don't preach. This may not be the time for a real deep conversation. Just say, "It's cool, I just don't feel like it," or "I don't like the taste." You can make your point without putting down your friends.

- Turn it into a joke. "Sure, let's drink. Then when I total my car, maybe my dad will buy me a new one—if I'm still alive."

- Take time out. If you're at a party, for example, go to the bathroom or step outside to clear your head. Then, if they ask again, you'll probably feel strong enough to say what you really mean.

■ If things are really getting out of hand, make yourself scarce. If you have a strong feeling you would rather be someplace else, go with it. You have a right to protect yourself; tomorrow you can tell your friends, "I had to get up early. You guys were out of it, so I just left."

■ Say what adults say. When the waiter comes around and offers a refill, an adult might say, "I'm good, thanks," and cover his or her glass with a hand. Sounds cool, doesn't it? It *is* cool, since it's a way of taking control and doing what *you* want to do.

GIVE IT A TRY

Peer pressure, about drinking or any other subject, isn't easy to resist. But in the end, the chances are, you will wind up with more and better friends if you do what you think is right. It is certainly worth trying.

See also: Advertising and Counteradvertising; Alcohol Abuse, The Risks of; Binge Drinking Among Teenagers; Underage Drinking

■ RECOVERY AND TREATMENT

Treating alcohol **abuse** (consequences of a drinking pattern that leads to intoxication or addiction causing behavioral problems) or alcoholism (a form of alcohol abuse in which the abuser is physically addicted to alcohol) can be a long, difficult process. Alcohol abusers often find that the hardest steps in the recovery process are the first ones: recognizing that they have a problem and deciding to fix it.

Many people who suffer from alcohol abuse do not want to admit that they are ill. Even when they do, they often hesitate to seek treatment, out of ignorance, fear, or a feeling of hopelessness. They are making a mistake. Alcohol abuse *can* be successfully treated. It takes time and effort, and there can be setbacks; but treatment has helped millions of alcoholics and alcohol abusers lead better lives.

Drinking can be unhealthy and dangerously habit-forming. You can—and should—avoid most of alcohol problems by learning sensible drinking behavior or by choosing to abstain (not drink at all). If you do not make a firm decision either way, you may find it very easy to fall into bad drinking habits—and very hard to pull yourself out.

Fact Or Fiction?

People can never recover from alcoholism.

Fact: It is true that many people, including those who follow the philosophy of Alcoholics Anonymous, believe that recovery from alcohol abuse is a life-long task. But don't misunderstand what they are saying. Millions of people in all walks of life have successfully confronted their alcohol problems and changed their behaviors. They and their families and friends are living better lives, thanks to self-help or formal treatment.

Since the time 80 years ago when people first began to think of alcohol abuse as a disease rather than a moral failing, doctors and therapists have been looking for ways to cure or treat the sufferers. It is a complicated process, involving several different levels of treatment. First of all, doctors must treat the physical harm that alcohol has done to the abuser's body. Then, if the abuser wants to stop drinking, doctors or clinics must deal with the difficult and sometimes dangerous symptoms of **withdrawal**.

The most difficult aspect to treat is the behavior itself. Since alcohol abuse, or alcoholism, does not have one simple cause, doctors can not inoculate people with a vaccine to prevent it. Nor can they prescribe an antibiotic to cure the behavior. So many different physical, emotional, and social factors can contribute to alcohol abuse, and they combine in different ways in each individual. Each of these factors may need to be dealt with separately:

- Physical cravings for alcohol
- Emotional problems that make people vulnerable to addictive behavior
- Family members, friends, or colleagues who drink a lot

■ Problems at home, school, or work that people may
want to escape

Health-care professionals and self-help innovators use many different methods to treat these factors, with different degrees of success.
Sometimes they argue among themselves about which method is best.
They even disagree on the crucial question: How can one measure
success in treating alcohol abuse?

With many diseases, such as measles or pneumonia, doctors try to
cure the patients, to help them recover completely and return to good
health. With other **chronic** (long-lasting) conditions, such as diabetes or
AIDS, doctors today cannot cure the underlying problem. Instead, they
try to keep the patients free of symptoms and help them to lead a normal life. Which kind of disease is alcohol abuse? Can anyone recover?

WHAT IS A RECOVERING ALCOHOLIC?

Nonaddictive alcohol abuse can sometimes be overcome by changes
in lifestyle, such as a move or a new job. It is much harder, however,
to deal with alcoholism itself. In fact, the majority of doctors and
therapists practicing in the United States today believe that no one
can ever completely recover from alcoholism.

A.A., or Alcoholics Anonymous, the largest and most influential
self-help movement in the field, has been promoting that belief since
it was founded in 1935. A.A. does accept that some "problem
drinkers" may recover but believes that those who are truly alcoholic
cannot. Most people under treatment for alcohol addiction are in programs inspired by A.A., and they are not aiming for complete recovery, or remission of symptoms. Instead, they call themselves
recovering alcoholics.

According to A.A., recovery is an ongoing process that continues
for the rest of the patient's life. A.A. members refer to themselves as
alcoholics even years after their last drink of alcohol. They know that
many nonalcoholics can handle moderate drinking, but they believe
that a recovering alcoholic is always in danger of abusing alcohol
again. They try to abstain from any form of alcohol. If they slip, as
they sometimes do, they are committed to returning to **sobriety** (non-
drinking). They also are committed to working on personal growth
and helping other alcoholics and others in need.

Some treatment professionals do not agree that alcoholism is incurable. They believe that by dealing with the problems that contribute to

addiction, and by learning new behaviors, alcoholics can be cured. Those experts define recovery as "a remission of symptoms over a certain period of time." In other words, the patient feels no cravings for alcohol for years at a time. The symptoms of abusive behavior may return in the future, like the symptoms of many other diseases. If they do, they can be treated once again.

Some individuals seem to recover without any formal treatment program. Sometimes a positive life change, such as a new job or the birth of a child, provides the incentive people need to face up to their drinking problem. And sometimes the opposite happens—a person realizes that alcohol is putting work, family, or even life itself at risk, and makes the decision to stop.

CAN THE ALCOHOLIC EVER DRINK SOCIALLY AGAIN?

This question has two parts. Experts disagree about the facts, but they also disagree about the message they want to convey to people who have not yet decided to seek treatment and to those who have been recovering for years.

Alcoholics Anonymous and the many other treatment programs it has inspired all give the question a firm answer: *no.* A.A.'s General Service Office writes, "All available medical testimony indicates that alcoholism is a progressive illness, that it cannot be cured in the ordinary sense of the term, but that it can be arrested through total abstinence from alcohol in any form." By progressive, they mean that the victims of this illness will always progress, or move along, from moderate drinking to addiction.

A.A. believes that alcoholics, by their very nature, have a tendency to abuse alcohol. Whether that tendency was inherited or learned from an alcoholic parent or acquired as a result of the ups and downs of life, A.A. believes that alcoholics are never able to get rid of their addiction completely.

A.A. advocates believe that the goal of abstinence is important, even if it is difficult to achieve. People may slip (by having a few drinks in a weak moment) or even have a relapse (by going back to problem drinking). But if they work toward abstinence as a goal, with the support of other A.A. members, the number and severity of their relapses can be limited.

Dr. Morris Chafetz, founding director of the National Institute for Alcohol Abuse and Alcoholism (NIAAA), wrote a book in 1976 called

Why Drinking Can Be Good for You. As the title makes clear, he is not a prohibitionist, and he believes that many people's lives are improved by moderate drinking. However, he writes, "Social drinking after severe alcoholism isn't such a good idea." Even though statistics show that some alcoholics can carry it off, "why they'd run the risk is beyond me. Alcohol is no necessity of life."

Some critics of the A.A. philosophy would go further. They say that even alcoholics can eventually go back to social drinking. As evidence, they cite the National Longitudinal Alcoholism Epidemiological Survey, which was completed in 1992. The survey looked at several thousand people who had been alcohol-dependent 20 years before and divided them into two groups—those who had been in treatment programs and those who had not.

The survey came up with surprising results. Twenty years after people first became dependent on alcohol, more than half of those who never even sought treatment were now able to drink without abuse. On the other hand, only 25 percent of those who had undergone treatment could now drink socially.

Of course, it is usually the people suffering the most from alcohol who enter treatment—or are forced into treatment programs by family, employer, or judge. That may explain why those who were treated were less likely to overcome alcoholism. And many of those who say they can now drink socially may not have really been alcoholics.

The goal of total abstinence may frighten some people away from treatment. Those people are sometimes more willing to try programs that provide the option of cutting back rather than quitting. If that doesn't work, such patients are usually willing to try full abstinence.

FORMS OF TREATMENT

At any one time, some 700,000 people in the United States are enrolled in treatment programs to deal with alcohol abuse, not counting self-help groups like A.A. Many different types of treatment are available. Some people use more than one of them over time, or even at the same time, to handle different aspects of their problems. The main variations are listed here.

Brief intervention

Brief intervention is a form of short-term therapy, aimed at changing behavior, that any trained social worker, educator, or physician can

DID YOU KNOW?

Percentage of Population Receiving Alcohol or Illicit-Drug Treatment

	Received Treatment in the Past Year[1]							
	Any Illicit Drug		Alcohol		Any Illicit Drug and Alcohol		Any Illicit Drug or Alcohol[2]	
Demographic Characteristic	2000	2001	2000	2001	2000	2001	2000	2001
Total	0.6	0.8	0.9	1.0	0.4	0.5	1.3	1.4
Age								
12–17	1.1	1.0	1.0	0.8	0.7	0.6	1.6	1.5
18–25	0.9	1.3	1.4	1.5	0.6	0.8	2.0	2.3
26 or Older	0.4	0.6	0.9		0.3	0.5	1.1	1.2
Gender								
Male	0.7	0.9	1.4	1.4	0.5	0.7	1.8	1.9
Female	0.5	0.6	0.5	0.6	0.3	0.4	0.8	0.9

Illicit drugs include marijuana/hashish, cocaine (including crack), heroin, hallucinogens, inhalants, or any prescription-type psychotherapeutic used nonmedically.

[1]"Received treatment" refers to treatment received in order to reduce or stop drug or alcohol use, or for medical problems associated with drug or alcohol use. It includes treatment received at any location, such as a hospital, at a rehabilitation facility (inpatient or outpatient), mental health center, emergency room, private doctor's office, self-help group, or prison/jail.

[2]Estimates include persons who received treatment specifically for alcohol or any illicit drug, as well as persons who received treatment but did not specify for what substance(s).

Source: National Household Survey on Drug Abuse, SAMHSA, Office of Applied Studies, 2000 and 2001.

perform. In it, the professionals tell problem drinkers, or potential problem drinkers, about the risks they are facing and let them know how to reduce or eliminate the risks. Sometimes they refer people to treatment programs.

Some colleges use "feedback surveys" for brief intervention. They ask students to fill out questionnaires about their own drinking, and to estimate how much the average student drinks. When the results are tabulated and sent back to the participants, many students who drink much more than the average seem to reevaluate their behavior and cut back. World Health Organization researchers in Australia reported in 1994 that even five minutes of advice to problem drinkers leads many of them to cut back by 25 percent.

Psychotherapy

In psychotherapy, a psychologist, social worker, or other trained professional works with patients to help relieve their emotional or behavioral problems, usually through discussions or counseling sessions.

Among the popular forms of psychotherapy for alcoholics are:

- **Motivational enhancement therapy.** The therapist actively encourages the patient to consider the effects of alcohol on his or her life. Together, they create and put into effect a practical plan to reduce or eliminate drinking.

- **Cognitive behavior skills therapy.** Once patients figure out the specific "triggers" that make them want to have a drink (time of day, place, person, or situation), the therapist helps them find different ways to respond to those triggers without drinking. For example, the patient might learn to say no when someone offers them a drink, or to call a friend rather than go out for a drink when their boss chews them out at work.

- **Individual psychotherapy.** The patient tries to understand the underlying emotional reasons for his or her drinking behavior. This usually takes longer than other types of therapy.

- **Group therapy.** A group of patients meet to discuss each other's problems. This can help people learn to communicate better with others and give them greater self-confidence.

- **Social skills therapy.** The therapist focuses on improving the patient's interpersonal skills in the hope that he or she becomes more successful in work and social life. That success might make the patient less prone to seek out alcohol as an escape.

- **Stress management.** The patient is taught ways to deal with pressure without drinking, such as muscle relaxing, biofeedback, or meditation.

- **Family therapy.** The therapist meets with the patient's family and gets them involved in the treatment process.

Self-help programs

For more than 70 years, Alcoholics Anonymous has been helping millions of people around the world deal with alcohol abuse and lead better lives. It has developed a loyal following and has inspired other groups to use similar methods to deal with drug abuse and other addictions.

The famous A.A. **Twelve-Step program** leads members through a series of stages with the goal of becoming "recovering alcoholics." The steps are designed to encourage people to face up to their problem and to the damage it has caused themselves and others. The program relies on a great deal of mutual help among members and a commitment to help others in the community as well.

Q & A

Question: Is Alcoholics Anonymous (A.A.) a Christian organization?

Answer: The group does not define itself as religious, and it accepts people of all religious faiths—and even those who adhere to no religion at all. Many present or former members say that critics of A.A. have exaggerated the religious aspect. However, the famous Twelve Steps does include several references to God "as we [each member] understands him." As a result, some people feel more comfortable attending other self-help groups that do not use the word *God*.

People who join and stick with A.A. share certain traits. They are more likely than the average alcoholic to have "hit bottom." They tend to be relatively extroverted, group-oriented, and able to discuss their problems with others. They also may be more religious and conservative than others.

However, A.A. may not work for everyone. In recent years, several other self-help organizations have emerged, some of them founded by former A.A. members. If A.A. doesn't work for an individual alcoholic, he or she may be able to fit into one of these groups.

Institutional programs

Many private and government agencies offer programs that combine medical treatment, psychotherapy, and social work to help alcoholics deal with their problems. They are often based on the Minnesota Model, a recovery program that was developed at the Hazelden Foundation near Center City, Minnesota, in the 1960s.

The original program included 28-day inpatient (live-in) care, combining **detoxification** and medical help, clinical psychology, and after-care support. It followed A.A.'s Twelve-Step recovery philosophy, and like A.A., it used recovering alcoholics as counselors. The Betty Ford Clinic in California is another influential example of the Minnesota Model.

A similar idea is used by halfway houses. These facilities are designed for alcoholics who have gone through detoxification but are not fully prepared to resume their normal lives without alcohol. Residents work in their normal careers during the day and participate in treatment in the evenings. The period of treatment can range from a few weeks to several months.

Family life

Whatever their philosophy, professionals in the field of alcohol abuse all stress how important the patient's family is, both in contributing to alcohol abuse and in helping to overcome it. They encourage patients to involve their families in treatment whenever possible.

One method is family therapy, in which the patient and his or her spouse, parents, or children meet on a regular basis with a therapist. The goals are to help the family understand the patient's problems and to find ways they can help provide a healthier or more supportive atmosphere. In other programs, the therapist might meet separately with the patient's family.

Another method is the one followed by Alanon and Alateen, offshoots of Alcoholics Anonymous. Alanon members are relatives, or sometimes close friends, of alcoholics. They meet in small groups on a regular basis to discuss how to deal with an alcoholic family member. Their primary goal is to prevent the patient's alcohol problems from overwhelming the family. But they also examine some of their own behavior that may be keeping the patient from facing up to his or her problems. Alateen is a similar program, with membership restricted to teenage relatives and friends of alcoholics.

Other treatments

Some therapists and patients prefer treatments that put less emphasis on analyzing or changing the patient's frame of mind. Instead, they prefer shorter-term treatments that focus more attention on the patient's body.

"Natural recovery" has become popular in recent years. It tries to address the patient's overall health, nutrition, and lifestyle needs. Some common treatment techniques are acupuncture, yoga, biofeedback, and nutritional supplements.

In "Faradic" aversion therapy, doctors try to get alcoholics to hate alcohol by administering electric shocks while they drink or see pictures of alcoholic beverages.

Some doctors favor certain medications in treating alcohol, often in combination with other treatments:

- **Naltrexone** and other **antagonists** can be used to take away the "high" that comes with alcohol. These drugs attach themselves to the same nerve cells in the brain that alcohol uses, pushing alcohol aside until it can be broken down in the liver.

- **Aversion drugs** such as **Antabuse** make patients feel sick to their stomachs as soon as they drink any alcohol. These drugs condition some patients to dislike alcohol.

- Doctors often prescribe sedatives and antidepressants to help relieve the emotional symptoms that cause some people to drink too much.

WHAT ARE THE NUMBERS?

The field of alcohol treatment is large, diverse, and controversial. Many treatment programs publish statistics claiming certain recovery rates, but they rarely report long-term follow-ups. As a result, experts in the field cannot agree on any firm statistics. However, they all agree that treatment has helped millions of alcohol abusers.

The two-year California Drug and Alcohol Treatment Assessment, reported in 1994, found that alcohol and drug use had declined 40 percent among those who underwent treatment. They were also one-third less likely to need hospitalization. Another national study found huge declines in the rate of arrests for criminals with records after they underwent treatment for alcoholism.

In a recent book, *The Facts About Drug Use*, Barry Stimmel, a noted physician and medical educator specializing in addiction research, concedes that many people do not believe alcohol treatments work. But this "pessimism," he writes, "is unwarranted."

Stimmel compares alcoholism with diabetes or asthma, which are also **chronic** (long-term) diseases that cannot be fully cured. Doctors know, he writes, that most patients with those diseases *occasionally* eat improperly or occasionally fail to take their medicine, and many of them suffer relapses as a result. Yet no one wants to abandon diabetes or asthma patients or eliminate the treatment programs for those diseases. In the same way, alcohol abuse treatments should be judged on whether they improve the patient's quality of life over the *long haul*. It would be foolish to give up on alcoholism treatment programs just because many alcoholics occasionally slip up.

NO REASON TO LOSE HOPE

Alcoholism *can* be treated successfully. Millions of people testify to having overcome their dependence, using any of a wide variety of treatments. Alcohol abusers willing to explore the available treatment options, and then devote time and hard work, have every reason to expect recovery and a better life.

See also: Alcohol and Disease; Peer Pressure and Alcohol; Self-Help Programs

FURTHER READING

Barry Stimmel. *Alcoholism, Drug Addiction, and the Road to Recovery: Life on the Edge.* New York: Haworth Medical Press, 2002.

■ RISK-TAKING

Behaviors that increase the probability of an unwanted event or potential loss. Elderly people know they may face health issues that are part of the normal aging process. Young people, in contrast, expect to enjoy robust good health, and most of them do. Unfortunately, some of them make behavior choices that put their health at risk. In fact, the major cause of death and chronic (long-term) illness among young people is risky behavior such as substance abuse, unsafe sex, and violence. That is why health educators try to focus on teenagers when dealing with risk-taking.

In the 21st century, every American 15-year-old can expect to live another 65 years, at least. And most of those years should be healthy and productive. Of course, you never know what dangers beyond your control will come tomorrow. But you should know that behavior choices that are within your control can make a big difference in your chances of living a long and healthy life.

While young people like to experiment, even "push the envelope" now and then, risky habits formed in the teenage years can later be difficult to break. The right choices now may make your future healthier and, most likely, more successful and fulfilling.

Alcohol abuse is on every list of major risk-taking behaviors. In fact, drinking too much and combining drinking with driving or sexual behaviors are near the top of every risk-taking list.

THE CENTERS FOR DISEASE CONTROL AND PREVENTION

The Centers for Disease Control and Prevention, located in Atlanta, Georgia, is often in the headlines for its role in monitoring and controlling sudden epidemics and new viruses. But this federally funded institution also has responsibilities for preventing chronic disease, through its Center for Chronic Disease Prevention.

Concerned about risk-taking among young people, the center set up the Youth Risk Behavior Surveillance System—YRBSS, for short—in 1990. By "surveillance," they weren't talking about spy satellites or telephone bugs. Instead, they have run repeated surveys, both nationwide and local, to ascertain how the country's teenagers were shaping up in terms of the following list of six major risk behaviors:

- Tobacco use
- Unhealthy dietary behaviors
- Inadequate physical activity
- Alcohol and other drug use
- Sexual behaviors that contribute to unintended pregnancy and sexually transmitted diseases, including HIV infection
- Behaviors that contribute to unintentional injuries and violence

These behaviors, the center said, were major contributors among teenagers to "the leading causes of death, disability, and social problems" (including heart disease, cancer, diabetes, and violent deaths). Furthermore, their reports show that the behaviors were "often established during childhood and early adolescence."

The center hoped that the surveys would uncover trends in young people's behavior, show the interconnections between different types of risk, highlight areas where education could improve behaviors, and monitor any improvements that education might bring.

YRBSS has conducted national, state, and local surveys of ninth-to12th-grade youngsters every two years since 1991. The program also runs special surveys of college students, high-risk kids in alternative high schools, and surveys of the entire population of 12- to 20-year-olds. A number of promising state and local health education programs have grown out of these surveys. The results of the various YRBSS surveys are available online.

CONSEQUENCES

When it finished analyzing the 2001 survey results, the YRBSS published a brief fact sheet that showed the connection between risk-taking behavior among high schools seniors and the leading causes of death for young people, as reported separately by the National Center of Health Statistics.

For people between 10 and 24 years old, the leading causes of death in 1999 were

- Motor vehicle crashes: 31 percent
- Homicide: 15 percent
- Suicide: 12 percent
- Other injury: 12 percent
- HIV infection: 1 percent
- All other causes: 19 percent

About 70 percent of all these tragically premature deaths were the result of injuries and violence, and alcohol was a major contributor to many of those deaths. In the 2001 survey, 30 percent of high school seniors reported "episodic heavy drinking" during the past month—having at least five drinks at a clip on at least five occasions. Also, 31 percent of seniors rode in a car with a drinking driver, 13 percent drove a car after drinking, and 4.9 percent had drunk alcohol on school property. A total of 33 percent were in physical fights, which are often alcohol-related.

The survey also tried to pin down the "age of initiation of risk behavior." In other words, how young are kids when risky behaviors first take place? With alcohol, 29 percent of kids had their first drink (not counting just a few sips) at 12 years old or younger.

As for combining alcohol and sex, more than one out of four sexually active students had used alcohol or drugs the last time they had sex. Much evidence shows that people who drink when they have sex tend to be careless about protecting themselves and their partner from unwanted pregnancy and sexually transmitted disease.

Nevertheless, optimists believe they have plenty of good news to focus on in the 2001 survey. Most of the risky behaviors have been declining among high school students since 1991. The trend has been uneven, but the overall figures are down. The exceptions are marijuana and cocaine use, which both increased.

For alcohol, the most significant change between 1991 and 2001 was a decline in the percentage of kids who rode with a driver who had been drinking. The incidence went from 39.9 to 30.7 percent.

The data is different for the older group—adults 25 and older. The leading causes of death for them were

- Cardiovascular (heart and blood vessel) disease: 41 percent

- Cancer: 24 percent

- Pulmonary (lung) disease: 4 percent

- Diabetes: 3 percent

- All others: 28 percent

Alcohol can be involved indirectly in some of these diseases, but the other risk factors have a more direct effect—tobacco, unhealthy diet (including too much sugar and fat), and inadequate physical activity all contribute to early death among adults.

America's high school seniors show early signs of the unhealthy patterns that harm adults. In the 2001 survey, 28 percent of high school seniors had smoked cigarettes in the past month, 79 percent were eating less than five servings of fruit and vegetables per day, 31 percent did not take part in even moderate physical activity, and 48 percent were not taking physical education at school.

ALTERNATIVES TO RISK-TAKING

In life, you can't avoid taking *some* risks. Even if you could, it would be a boring life, especially for adventurous teenagers.

Educators concerned about unhealthy risk-taking, however, have talked up the idea of *healthy* risk-taking as an alternative. In her book *The Romance of Risk: Why Teenagers Do the Things They Do,* adolescent psychotherapist Lynn Ponton suggests alternatives that might interest kids who are taking some dangerous risks. For example, kids involved in bullying or gang violence might want to take on the emotional risk of seeking out new friends or moving to a different school; those behaviors probably take a lot more courage than ganging up on a smaller kid.

As for alcohol- and drug-abusing teens, the book suggests that they look into the "extreme physical and emotional thrills" of white-water rafting, rock climbing, and other vigorous sports. The key is to redefine "risk" as "challenge." What challenge do you meet, the writer asks, when you guzzle down five or six beers and jump behind the steering wheel?

Many schools around the United States and Canada have begun "alternatives to risk-taking" programs, built around after-school recreational, educational, and community service programs. Other schools have used that term as the title of class units that teach kids how to resist friends or classmates who try to pressure them into taking risks they do not want to take. Whichever alternatives they offer, these schools recognize that the old slogan "Just say no" may not be enough to convince today's kids.

BE SMART

Taking risks is part of life. Taking *harmful* risks when sensible alternatives are available is a part of life that smart teenagers avoid.

See also: Alcohol Abuse, The Risks of; Alcohol and Disease; Alcohol and Violence; Drinking and Driving; Effects on the Body; Sexual Behavior and Alcohol

■ RISKS AND ALCOHOL

See: Alcohol Abuse, The Risks of

■ SELF-HELP PROGRAMS

A series of steps or services that help overcome a problem. Alcohol **abuse** can be a very sad topic, but one inspiring chapter in the story is the self-help movement created by alcoholics and their families. Through hard work, courage, and initiative, they have developed new ways of dealing with alcoholism and other addictive behaviors. They have given new hope and confidence to millions of people.

HISTORY OF ALCOHOLICS ANONYMOUS

The story of A.A., or **Alcoholics Anonymous**, began in Akron, Ohio, in 1935. The founders were "Bill W.," a stockbroker, and "Dr. Bob S.," a surgeon, both of whom had been severe alcoholics.

Bill had become sober through his membership in the Oxford Group, a Christian organization that tried to bring spiritual values into daily life. Some of the techniques of A.A., and much of its Twelve-Step philosophy came from the Oxford Group. But the core idea that alcoholism should be considered a disease came from Dr. William Silkworth, a physician to whom Bill had often gone for **detoxification** treatment.

The two founders, Bill W. and Dr. Bob, decided early on that only alcoholics themselves could help one another overcome their specific problems. They spread their message among other alcoholics and helped organize groups of like-minded alcoholics into small self-help groups. By 1939, when Bill published *Alcoholics Anonymous*, a book-length guide to recovery with successful case histories, about 100 members had become sober in three different cities.

The group filled a desperate need for treatment; its message of hope proved appealing. A.A. has not stopped growing since. By 1951, a "General Service Conference" was formed to provide central services and publish books and pamphlets for members of the groups and interested outsiders.

In 1939, family groups began to form as an outgrowth of A.A. Relatives of alcoholics got together to discuss the problems that alcoholism brings to the families and friends of alcoholics. In 1951, Bill W.'s wife cofounded Al-Anon to coordinate the several dozen groups that had formed in the United States and abroad. By 1997, Al-Anon Family Groups, the coordinating body, claimed that 30,000 groups exist in 115 countries.

Alateen, devoted to teenage family members and friends of alcoholics, was founded in 1957. Like Al-Anon, it adheres to the

Twelve-Step philosophy, and its groups function in accordance with the A.A. model.

A.A. TODAY

Alcoholics Anonymous, the pioneer organization in treating alcohol abuse, now claims more than one million members in the United States, organized into more than 50,000 self-supporting local groups. A.A.'s affiliates (associated groups) around the world have another million members. Millions of past members have also recovered in whole or in part as a result of A.A.

According to a 2001 membership survey (published by the A.A. General Service Conference), men outnumber women by two to one. All age groups are represented, though only one out of nine members is under 30 years old. More than one-third are married, another third are single, and about one-quarter are divorced. The group is racially and economically diverse, although a large majority of members are whites.

The average member attends two meetings a week. Most important, the survey reports that members have been sober for an average of seven years. The large majority of members have also taken advantage of other forms of treatment or counseling, often while attending A.A. group meetings.

The group describes itself as "a fellowship of men and women who share their experience, strength and hope with each other that they may solve their common problem and help others to recover from alcoholism." Members run and fund their own groups, along guidelines provided by the national organization. Membership is free, and tradition ensures that anyone who wants to become sober is welcomed.

A.A. has continued its practice of strict anonymity—people are known on a first-name basis only—even though alcoholism is no longer considered shameful by most people. In today's world, A.A. says, anonymity helps to keep the organization free of power struggles and corruption. Any group leadership positions are rotated among the members.

The basic treatment philosophy of A.A. is that "an alcoholic who no longer drinks has an exceptional faculty for 'reaching' and helping an uncontrolled drinker." In others words, the best person to help an alcoholic recover is a recovering alcoholic. Toward that end, the group aims to provide a "sponsor" to each new member. The sponsor is available at all times to share his or her experiences, provide moral support, and help the "sponsee" overcome any problems that could lead him or her back to alcohol abuse. The 2001 survey found that 78

DID YOU KNOW?

The Twelve Steps

Alcoholics Anonymous recommends the Twelve Steps listed below as a guide for individuals trying to overcome alcoholism. Many other self-help groups now use similar steps in their recovery programs.

1. We admitted we were powerless over alcohol—that our lives had become unmanageable.
2. Came to believe that a Power greater than ourselves could restore us to sanity.
3. Made a decision to turn our will and our lives over to the care of God as we understood Him.
4. Made a searching and fearless moral inventory of ourselves.
5. Admitted to God, to ourselves and to another human being the exact nature of our wrongs.
6. Were entirely ready to have God remove all these defects of character.
7. Humbly asked Him to remove our shortcomings.
8. Made a list of all persons we had harmed, and became willing to make amends to them all.
9. Made direct amends to such people wherever possible, except when to do so would injure them or others.
10. Continued to take personal inventory and when we were wrong promptly admitted it.
11. Sought through prayer and meditation to improve our conscious contact with God, as we understood Him, praying only for knowledge of His will for us and the power to carry that out.
12. Having had a spiritual awakening as the result of these steps, we tried to carry this message to alcoholics and to practice these principles in all our affairs.

percent of members had a sponsor and that 71 percent had gotten a sponsor within 90 days of joining up.

Members are supposed to be guided by the "Twelve Steps" to recovery. The first step, which is said to be the most difficult, is for alcoholics to admit that they are "powerless over alcohol." In other words, they cannot beat the problem without help from a "Power greater than ourselves," which A.A. defines as "God as we understand Him."

Several steps revolve around members taking a "moral inventory," trying to understand their faults and the way they have hurt other people. They then try to "make amends" with the people they have harmed. Finally, they make a commitment to spread the message to other alcoholics and to conduct themselves according to these principles in the future.

Someone who decides to try A.A., or has been sent to A.A. by a treatment program, usually attends orientation meetings, aided by a guide who sometimes becomes the sponsor. The new member is then encouraged to make a commitment to attend a certain number of meetings, often 90 meetings in 90 days, even if they must put aside other personal commitments to do so. In most cities, there are groups meeting every day.

Even for those who find the meetings helpful, it may take some time before a new member admits to having a problem and makes the famous statement, "My name is _____, and I am an alcoholic." In fact, the earliest stage is probably crucial to success within the group. Success seems to depend in part on how accepting the group is.

Many A.A. members are firmly convinced that they would not have been able to overcome their problems without A.A. The acceptance and support they get from other members made it easier for them to adopt new ways of thinking about themselves and new, more healthy behaviors.

A.A., however, is not necessarily the best treatment for every individual. People who attend a few meetings and drop out should not consider themselves failures. It may be that another A.A. group, or a different self-help program, or another type of treatment altogether, may be more to their liking. Besides, even "dropouts" can benefit from the stories they hear and the literature they read while attending A.A.

AL-ANON

Al-Anon was founded by family members of A.A. members, and follows A.A.'s Twelve-Step philosophy; however, the two groups are not formally connected, and Al-Anon is run independently both on the local and national levels.

Al-Anon members consider alcoholism to be a "family disease." When one member of a family is a serious alcoholic, everyone else suffers to a degree. Families often may be harmed in practical ways, when the alcoholic fails to carry his or her weight financially or as a good spouse or parent. Sometimes the emotional toll is even higher, with fear, anger, resentment, and loneliness taking over the home.

Too often, family members also may be victimized by violence at the hands of the alcoholic individual. Members are encouraged to learn how to protect themselves and, if necessary, to involve the authorities. Al-Anon believes that no one is helped when families try to protect violent alcoholics from the consequences of their behavior.

The purpose of Al-Anon is to allow members to help one another by sharing their stories and successes in dealing with their common problems. They believe this process helps them change their own unhealthy attitudes and behaviors that result from their relative or friend's alcoholism.

Al-Anon believes that the alcoholic must work towards his or her own recovery. But the family can help avoid behaviors that "enable" the alcoholic to remain stuck in his or her disease. For example, they must stop making excuses for the alcoholic and must look out for the family's interest even at the expense of the alcoholic, if he or she is uncooperative.

Some 85 percent of Al-Anon members are women, most often the wives of alcoholics. They tend to be a bit older than the average A.A. member but otherwise represent a cross-section of people. Their alcoholic family member is not necessarily a member of A.A., and may not even be in treatment. In fact, Al-Anon's literature insists that "no situation is really hopeless and that it is possible to find contentment and even happiness, whether the alcoholic is drinking or not."

As is the case with A.A., the majority of Al-Anon members have participated in other counseling or treatment programs to help deal with their family's alcoholism problems. Al-Anon meetings help reinforce the benefits of those programs.

ALATEEN

Teenagers with an alcoholic family member (who is usually a parent) experience all the problems of other family members, and perhaps a few more of their own. Adolescents should be able to rely on parents for advice and support as they learn to become adults. Instead, many teen children of alcoholics get little or no support from the alcoholic parent. They often get less support than they need even from the non-alcoholic parent, who may be preoccupied.

Kids tend to care very much about what their friends and school-mates think. Frequently embarrassed by their alcoholic parent's behavior, they may even withdraw from friends; angry or frustrated, they sometimes misbehave in and out of school.

Alateen, like its parent-group Al-Anon, takes many of its ideas from A.A., including anonymity, the Twelve Steps, sponsors, and the idea of mutual help among people sharing the same problems. Every Alateen group has an adult sponsor who is a member of Al-Anon.

There are now some 2,700 Alateen groups meeting around the world. The average age of members is 13; 62 percent are girls.

OTHER SELF-HELP GROUPS

Over the years, former members of A.A. who felt that the organiza-tion did not meet their particular needs, and other people who dis-agreed with parts of the A.A. philosophy, have created several other types of self-help groups. None of them has grown nearly as large as A.A., but they can be a useful alternative for some people.

Women for Sobriety was founded in 1976, when the modern fem-inist movement was in full swing. Its members believe that women's recovery needs are different from men's and are not fully recognized by A.A. They agree with A.A.'s disease model of alcoholism and its goal of **abstinence**, and like A.A. their "New Life" program includes a system of levels (steps) and statements of principles. But they stress individual responsibility for change rather than reliance on a "higher power." The group boasts several hundred groups in six countries.

Secular Organizations for Sobriety has been in existence since 1986. It is designed "for those alcoholics or drug addicts who are uncomfortable with the spiritual content" of A.A. and similar groups. They claim member groups in every state and some foreign countries. Like A.A., they advocate abstinence.

SMART (Self Management and Recovery Training, founded in 1994) is another nonspiritual self-help organization with a few hundred member groups. It rejects the disease model of alcoholism and does not advocate lifetime membership. They offer online groups as well.

Moderation Management was founded in 1993. It is the only alco-holism self-help organization that believes in moderate drinking as a possible goal—but only after the new member goes through a period of abstinence. It is designed for "problem drinkers" rather than alcoholics, especially drinkers in the "beginning stage" who have not progressed to serious alcohol **dependency**.

FROM PAIN TO INSPIRATION

Thanks to the success of Alcoholics Anonymous, self-help groups have proliferated (spread widely) in communities all across the United States. Together they offer information, encouragement, and inspiration to millions of people.

See also: Children of Alcoholics; Law and Drinking, The; Recovery and Treatment

FURTHER READING

Alcoholics Anonymous: The Story of How Many Thousands of Men and Women Have Recovered from Alcoholism. New York: Alcoholics Anonymous World Services, 2001.

Joseph Nowinski. *The Twelve-Step Facilitation Handbook: A Systematic Approach to Early Recovery from Alcoholism and Addiction.* San Francisco, CA: Jossey-Bass, 1998.

Margi Trapani. *Inside a Support Group: Help for Teenage Children of Alcoholics.* New York: Rosen Publishing Group, 1997.

■ SEXUAL BEHAVIOR AND ALCOHOL

Drinking and sex have one thing in common. They can be safe when done wisely and carefully. But if you do either one foolishly, you can get into trouble. And if you do them foolishly at the same time, you double your risk.

Drinking and sex are connected in another way. Some people deliberately use alcohol to overcome shyness and initiate social or sexual contact with an appropriate partner. Others believe that alcohol increases their sexual drive or performance or at least makes them feel more relaxed and able to respond to their partner.

Combining sex and alcohol has a big negative side too. Alcohol may lead many people to give in to sex when they really want to say no. Sex and alcohol also may lead to unwanted pregnancy, **sexually transmitted diseases (STDs)**, violence, and rape, and can cause guilt, fear, and broken relationships. The problem is separating the good from the bad.

IS ALCOHOL AN APHRODISIAC?

According to research, **aphrodisiacs** (foods or drinks that increase romantic or sexual desire) do not really exist, although you could spend a bundle on the Internet buying products that promise to do the trick. Yet for many people, one or two drinks have a relaxing effect, distracting them from their worries and loosening the control centers in their brains. As a result, they may feel more tender and loving, at the right time and place, and more aware of their natural sexual feelings.

On the other hand, as people continue drinking, the opposite effect kicks in. Sex involves two people, and therefore needs sensitivity and attention, which usually go out the window when people are intoxicated. And if you keep on drinking, you can become unable to perform—even if you can stay awake. As one expert put it, "Heavy drinkers have lousy sex lives."

Alcohol can stimulate sex in another, more sinister, way. Some people believe that alcohol makes them more virile and desirable. Since they are often mistaken, this belief can lead to misunderstandings and even serious trouble for others.

Fact Or Fiction?

Alcohol can improve a man's sexual performance.

Fact: This one is somewhat true, but mostly false. A small amount of alcohol may help some men relax and feel sociable, which is helpful in any kind of romantic or sexual situation. But if a man has several drinks, his ability to do any physical task, including sex, starts to decline rapidly. Habitual heavy drinking can lead to impotence and even sterility.

SEXUAL COERCION

Sexual coercion, in which one person forces another person to have sexual relations against his or her will, can take many forms. Its most extreme form is rape, in which one person forces the other to have sexual relations against his or her will.

DID YOU KNOW?

According to the U.S. Department of Justice, alcohol plays an especially large role in sexual crimes. This table shows the percent of criminal offenders who seemed to be under the influence of alcohol or drugs during their crimes.

Percent of Crimes Involving Alcohol Abuse

	All Crimes of Violence	Rape or Sexual Assault*
Total crimes	100.0%	100.0%
Under influence of drugs or alcohol	28.1	43.6
Under the influence of alcohol	17.6	31.7
Under the influence of drugs	4.6	5.4
Under the influence of both		
drugs and alcohol	4.6	6.5
Not on alcohol or drugs	28.1	33.4
Don't know or not ascertained	43.8	23.0

* Includes verbal threats of rape and sexual assault.

Source: National Criminal Victimization Survey, Bureau of Justice Statistics, 2001.

Rape is a violent crime that is rightly punished by long prison sentences. It can inflict terrible emotional damage on its victims, as well as serious practical consequences such as unwanted pregnancy (a woman carrying the rapist's child) or sexually transmitted disease. Alcohol use is strongly connected with rape, both statistically (a high percentage of rapists drink before the rape) and psychologically (alcohol may "prepare" the rapist for the crime).

Coercion also includes less extreme crimes such as sexual assault, where one person physically forces attentions on another person. As in the case of rape, sexual assault often involves alcohol, according to *Alcohol Health and Research World*. In 1993 the journal reported studies showing that in one-third to three-quarters of all rapes and sexual assaults, the attacker or the victim—and often both—have been drinking. The proportion is highest for particularly violent rapes.

Some male rapists believe that women who drink are signaling that they are available for sex. In fact, a survey reported by the U.S. Department of Health and Human Services in 1992 found that 39 percent of high school boys and 18 percent of girls agreed with that statement. But this old myth is not true. (If people put themselves in the victim's shoes, they would think differently).

It is not surprising that many victims of sexual coercion have been drinking themselves. Women become intoxicated more quickly after drinking the same amount of alcohol as a man. Once intoxicated, they may miss warning signs that they are in danger and once they do understand, they may be unable to communicate their disapproval forcefully enough.

When sexual attacks begin, victims who have been drinking may not have the mental and physical resources they need to fight off their attackers. After the rape is over, they may feel shame that they drank enough to put themselves in danger, or they may not remember enough of the details to be sure of what really happened. But when victims regret their own actions, it does not excuse the rapist or the crime. It only highlights that taking advantage of someone against her will is a cowardly act as well as a criminal one.

Acquaintance rape, where the victim knew the perpetrator before the attack took place, is often associated with alcohol. On college campuses, according to a 2001 Justice Department report, nearly 90 percent of victims of rape or attempted rape on campuses personally knew the offender. In most of those, both the attacker and the victim had been drinking.

UNINTENDED SEX

People change their minds all the time, about sex as much as any other thing. Two "consenting adults" might have every intention of engaging in sexual relations on a particular occasion, yet something gets in the way (for example, drinking too much), and the plans fall through. But in other cases, one or both of the parties may have no intention of having sex, but under the influence of alcohol they change their minds.

It is not surprising that alcohol, the original "disinhibitor" that allows people to do things they wouldn't do sober, can lead to unplanned sex. A 2002 study by the Kaiser Family Foundation found that 29 percent of people between 15 and 17 years old admit that they are more sexually active than they plan to be due to alcohol and drug use. The number rises to 37 percent for the 18 to 24 age group.

A 1999 college survey reported by the Harvard University School of Public Health found that binge drinkers (men who drink five or more alcoholic drinks at one time, and women who drink four or more) were five times more likely to have unplanned sex as other students.

Unintended sex is usually unprepared and unprotected sex as well. It is often unappreciated too, the morning after. When sober, most people say that sex is important enough for them to carefully choose the time, place, and partner ahead of time. Under the influence of alcohol, however, people are less likely to stick to their own standards.

UNPROTECTED SEX

To state the obvious: Sex can have serious consequences. A woman of childbearing age (usually from the teenage through the middle-age years) is at risk of becoming pregnant from a single, brief sexual encounter, unless she or her partner deliberately uses birth control. Also, anyone who is careless about sex is at risk of getting a sexually transmitted disease, no matter what type of sexual behavior is involved.

Common sense suggests that people who are drinking when they have sex are less likely to use protection, since alcohol weakens the rational control centers of the brain. However, the evidence from surveys is not clear. One study published in 2003 in the journal *Perspectives on Sexual and Reproductive Health* found that teens were just as likely to use condoms after drinking alcohol than when they have not been drinking. However, other studies show that men and women who drink and also use drugs are much less likely than others to use condoms during sex. In those cases, it is hard to prove that alcohol is the cause of unprotected sex. A careless disregard for risk may cause both behaviors.

Unwanted pregnancies

As everyone knows, the only guaranteed way to avoid unwanted pregnancy is to abstain from sex. If you choose to practice **abstinence** before marriage, remember that it is easier to stick with your principles if you remain sober. The more you drink, the less likely you are to remain true to your values.

The next most effective methods available to women to keep from becoming pregnant are birth control pills, shots, patches, or skin implants, which prevent ovulation (the release of eggs in the womb), and intrauterine devices (IUD), which block sperm from reaching the egg. None of these methods requires protective action at the time of sex, so alcohol does not increase the risk of pregnancy.

Many women, especially young women, rely on condoms as their first line of defense—which means they must rely on men to use condoms too. To be fully effective, condoms have to be used correctly. For example, people should only use unopened condoms from an unbroken package that has not passed its expiration date. They should not use any petroleum-based lubricant, such as Vaseline, which can break down the latex in the condom. They should leave room at the tip of the condom to collect semen and keep it from seeping out the top. They should keep the condom on after withdrawal, and they should throw it away after use. Also, according to most experts, they should use latex rather than lambskin condoms to protect against sexually transmitted diseases (STDs), although both types are equally effective in preventing pregnancy. Now, do you think you can remember and carry out all these instructions after having several drinks?

Sexually transmitted diseases (STDs)
Until the invention of antibiotics early in the twentieth century, STDs were recognized as a very serious threat to public health (they were called "venereal diseases" in those days). Syphilis, perhaps the most feared of the STDs, often led to insanity and death.

The introduction of penicillin in the 1940s seemed to promise a world free of STDs. Before too long, however, the bacteria and other organisms that cause the most common STDs started developing resistance to penicillin and other antibiotic drugs. Today, it takes larger and larger doses of antibiotics to knock out a syphilis or gonorrhea infection. Even worse, the medical profession soon learned that serious virus infections, such as herpes and hepatitis B and C, were being widely spread through sexual contact.

The list of common STDs has grown with time. The world has become a smaller place; tiny disease-bearing organisms from all over the world seem to travel as easily as the most restless jet setter. The list includes chlamydia (which can cause sterility), fungus infections, yeast infections, venereal lice, and human papilloma virus (which can cause cervical cancer).

In 1981 a new STD surfaced—acquired immunodeficiency syndrome, or **AIDS**. Though it can also be passed from one person to another through contact with infected blood, most patients have been infected during sexual activity.

Every year about 15 million new cases of STDs occur in the United States. The two main risk factors that help spread STDs so widely are unprotected sex and multiple sexual partners.

Unprotected sex allows the exchange of infected body fluids, like semen or traces of blood. An infected individual may have enough bacteria or virus particles in those body fluids to infect the healthy partner after just one sexual contact. This is possible even if the infected partner does not show any symptoms of the disease. Almost any type of sexual activity between unprotected partners has the potential of spreading STDs.

The chances of transmission are increased if either partner has a sore or skin infection to begin with, or if his or her skin is chafed or torn during sex. The risk of transmission during unprotected sex is 30 percent for herpes, and up to 50 percent for gonorrhea.

The most effective protection against STDs during sex is a latex condom. Other birth control methods, such as pills, IUDs, diaphragms, and spermicidal creams, do nothing to protect against STDs. Lambskin condoms have tiny holes big enough for HIV, the virus that causes AIDS, to pass through.

Since alcohol can impair people's judgment and self-control, people who have been drinking often neglect to use condoms or fail to use them properly. Alcohol may play an even greater role in the other major risk factor for STDs—multiple sex partners.

One study of young people aged 14–22, reported in the journal *Family Planning Perspectives* in 2001, found that 61 percent of boys and 44 percent of girls who drank or used drugs during their last sexual encounter had had multiple partners in the previous three months, as compared with only 32 percent of boys and 14 percent of girls who had been sober the last time they had sex. Just by the law of averages, the more partners an individual has, the more likely he or she is to encounter an STD.

Q & A

Question: Do I need to practice safe sex if my partner has never had sex before?

Answer: If both you *and* your partner have never had sex of any kind with any other person, you will both remain free of STDs. But anyone who agrees to have sex with you may have agreed to have sex with another person. In other words, it really makes sense to play it safe—don't let alcohol cloud your judgment: Abstain from sex or limit your partners, and *practice safe sex every time.*

HIV and AIDS

In 1981, doctors in several American cities detected an epidemic of a new disease they named AIDS, or Acquired Immunodeficiency Disease. Two years later researchers discovered the organism that caused the disease—the human immunodeficiency virus (HIV)—and they showed that it could be easily passed along during sexual contact.

People can get infected with HIV through other means as well, such as sharing hypodermic needles or getting a transfusion of infected blood, but the large majority of victims have acquired the virus during sexual activity. If one unprotected partner has HIV, the other has a 1–4 percent chance of getting the virus during each sexual act. The risk depends on the particular act they perform.

HIV does its damage by harming, and eventually destroying, the body's immune system. This process can take several years to develop, but once the immune system is damaged the body becomes more vulnerable to dangerous and fatal illnesses such as pneumonia, painful nerve inflammations, liver disease, and cancer. By 2002, according to the Centers for Disease Control, AIDS had killed 501,000 Americans.

It took some 15 years before drugs were developed that could control AIDS. Drugs discovered in the 1990s have been successful in holding off fatal complications in most patients, and AIDS deaths began to decline in the United States. But these drugs are expensive, and they have not been available for most AIDS victims in poor countries. In 2002, according to the Joint United Nations Program on HIV/AIDS, more than three million people in countries all over the world died of AIDS, bringing total deaths to 28 million in just 21 years. Some five million new people were infected with HIV in 2002, 40,000 of them in the United States.

New strains of HIV have begun to appear that the medicines cannot reach. In any case, these drugs only help people who are already sick; so far, no one has been able to make a vaccine that can be given to healthy people to keep the virus away.

When the epidemic first broke out in the United States, most of the victims were gay (homosexual) men. That has changed a long time ago, as the virus spread into wider communities. In most of the world, most people with AIDS are straight (heterosexual), and about half are women.

Due to the rise of AIDS, unprotected sex is far more dangerous than ever before. There has never been a better reason to use a latex condom. This is true for heterosexuals as well as for homosexuals. It is just as true for women and girls as for men and boys. It does not matter what part of the country you come from, what neighborhood you live in, or what race or ethnic group you belong to.

The best way to keep free of HIV is to abstain from sex. The next best way is to practice safe sex. That means you should:

- use good judgment in choosing sex partners;
- keep the number of partners to a minimum;
- avoid any activity that might cause skin tears or abrasions; and
- always use a condom, no matter what act you perform.

This is where alcohol comes in. Alcohol, especially in large quantities, can influence people to break every one of the rules of safe sex. It can lead you to have sex when you did not intend to or do not even want to; it impairs your judgment in choosing a partner; a pattern of alcohol abuse can lead to multiple partners; the lack of mental control can cause you to "forget" to use a condom; and the lack of physical control could make skin tears and abrasions more likely.

A study at Louisiana State University in 2003 suggested an even more direct link between alcohol and HIV. When alcohol is present in the bloodstream, researchers found, the body may be more susceptible to being infected by HIV during sexual contact.

Everyone knows that kids can make mistakes. It is part of growing up. But getting AIDS is too high a price to pay for the mistake of carelessly mixing drink and sex. Wouldn't you agree?

A DANGEROUS MIX

Drinking and driving is such a dangerous combination that it is against the law. Drinking and sex is not against the law, but don't be fooled—it can be very dangerous too.

Mature, experienced adults can usually handle the risks. Teenagers experimenting with these powerful behaviors very often can't. Smart kids do not allow social pressure and opportunity to take them down this path before they are ready. What's the rush?

See also: Alcohol and Violence; Binge Drinking Among Teenagers; Drinking on College Campuses; Risk-Taking

FURTHER READING

Faith Hickman Brynie. *101 Questions About Sex and Sexuality*. Brookfield, CT: Twenty-First Century Books, 2003.

Mary E. Williams, Tamara L. Roleff, eds. *Sexual Violence: Opposing Viewpoints*. San Diego, CA: Greenhaven Press, 1997.

■ TAKING RISKS

See: Risk-Taking

■ TEENAGERS AND ALCOHOL

See: Binge Drinking Among Teenagers; Children of Alcoholics; Choices, Responsible; Drinking and Driving; Peer Pressure and Alcohol; Underage Drinking

■ TREATMENT

See: Recovery and Treatment; Self-Help Programs

■ UNDERAGE DRINKING

Underage drinking means the consumption of alcoholic beverages by anyone under 21. That is the minimum age in all 50 states to legally purchase alcohol, whether at retail stores, restaurants, or bars.

Some states have exceptions built into the law; for example, some married people under 21 may purchase alcohol. In 19 states, younger people may legally drink in certain limited circumstances, such as in their home with parents. In fact, parents are almost never prosecuted in any state for serving alcohol to their own children in their own home.

Some experts recommend lowering the drinking age to 18 or 19, especially in those states that raised it in the late 1980s. They note that the legal drinking age is lower in every other country in the world—16, 18, or 20 in most democratic countries. The ages in Canadian provinces vary between 18 and 19.

Dr. Ruth Engs, Professor of Applied Health Sciences at Indiana University, is one of those who favors reducing the legal drinking age and teaching responsible drinking in schools. She claims that one of the reasons many young people drink irresponsibly is that "drinking is seen by these youth as an enticing 'forbidden fruit,' a 'badge of rebellion against authority,' and a symbol of adulthood." She points to the experiment of national **Prohibition** in the 1920s, which promoted widespread disrespect for law.

On the other side of the debate, those who support the current legal age point out that Prohibition did in fact reduce the total amount of drinking and alcohol abuse. They also claim that the age-18 drinking limit helps keep down the death toll from drunk driving car crashes. They say that the increase in the legal age to 21, which many states carried out the late 1980s, was the primary reason for a dramatic decline in teenage drunken driving crashes. That decline translates to 1,000 fewer teenage deaths per year. Putting the age back down to 18 or 19, they fear, would send the wrong signal to the nation's kids.

Whichever camp is right, both agree that the laws are not always strictly enforced. In a 2002 law enforcement campaign in Montgomery County, Maryland, 38 percent of underage decoys were able to purchase alcohol. Other states have reported similar findings.

WHO ARE THE YOUNG DRINKERS?

Despite the law, underage drinking is widespread. At every age level, across regional, gender, and ethnic lines, there are at least some kids who engage in casual drinking or occasional binges, and some who are alcoholics. By the time kids reach the 18 to 20 age group, alcohol behavior does not differ much from that of adults.

The National Household Survey on Drug Abuse (NHSDA) questions a typical sample of Americans every year about drug and alcohol use among their family members. They total up the results by age, gender, race, and other categories and publish them in tables and in colorful charts. The alcohol-use charts are very dramatic. They look like familiar pictures of the Rock of Gibraltar—a sharp rise on the left (representing the underage groups) up to a peak at age 21, followed by a gradual drop-off in the later years.

Twenty-year-olds, the last "underage" group, are among the country's heaviest drinkers. To be precise, the 2001 survey reports that 55.7 percent of all 20-year-olds had drunk at least one alcoholic beverage during the previous month. Not only did the majority drink, but 38.2 percent (nearly four out of ten) were binge drinkers—they had drunk five or more drinks on at least one occasion that month—and 14.5 percent (one in seven) were heavy drinkers, having five or more drinks on five or more days that month.

The younger age groups drink a lot less alcohol. Only 2.6 percent of 12-year-olds, the youngest group counted in the survey, drank any alcohol in the previous month, and only one in a thousand of them were heavy drinkers. But the numbers rise quickly from that low base each subsequent year. For example, slightly more than 1 percent of 14-year-olds are heavy drinkers, as are 2 percent of 15-year-olds, 4 percent of 16-year-olds, 7 percent of 17-year-olds, and fully ten percent of 18-year-olds.

As for the gender breakdown, almost the exact same number (17 percent) of boys and girls in the 12- to 17-year-old age group drank at least once during the month. The girls did drink less, although the overall level of intoxication may have been the same, since girls need fewer drinks to get drunk. Only 1.9 percent of girls in the 12- to 17-year-old age group were considered heavy drinkers, as compared with 3.1 percent of the boys.

The racial or ethnic breakdown among the 12- to 17-year-olds showed more dramatic differences: African-American kids drank the least, followed by Asian Americans, Hispanic Americans, Caucasians, and Native Americans. The heavy drinking category included Caucasians (3.0 percent), Hispanic Americans (2.1 percent), Asian Americans (1.3 percent), and African Americans (0.7 percent).

Some educators and parents are shocked at these large numbers. However, drinking was even more common in the recent past. The National Institute on Drug Abuse has been following drinking trends among high school seniors since 1980. In 1980, 72 percent of seniors reported using alcohol during the past month, and 41.2 percent had binged. By 2000, the numbers had fallen to 50 and 30 percent, respectively. Similar declines occurred among boys and girls, whites and blacks. Other researchers have found similar patterns. While alcohol and drug abuse seemed to decline among young people in the 1980s, the decline continued at a slower pace in the 1990s.

THE RISKS OF RAPID PROGRESSION

When people ask what you hope to be when you grow up, no one will answer "an alcoholic." But every year, teenagers who thought they could handle a few drinks fall into the trap.

Every year, about 250,000 teenagers enroll in treatment programs for alcohol abuse. Unfortunately, experts believe that for every kid who signs up, several others need treatment and don't get it. Nationwide, the National Institute for Alcohol Abuse and Alcoholism estimates that between 5.2 and 5.5 million teenager abuse alcohol.

Most of the kids entering treatment do not show the severe physical effects that long-term adult alcoholics do, but they are definitely addicted. The therapists who screen kids for addiction depend a lot on behavioral signs, such as how often the patient gets drunk, or how he or she manages relationships with others.

Researchers have found that the younger kids are when they start to drink, the greater their risk for rapid progression to alcohol **abuse** and addiction. In other words, it takes younger kids less time to get addicted than older kids or adults. In 2003 the American Journal of Psychiatry published a review of many recent studies showing that adolescents may be more prone to alcohol and drug addiction, since their brains change more rapidly in response to a new stimulus (such as alcohol).

When kids drink heavily, even if they avoid actual addiction, they may be damaging their brain, according to other recent research. A 2002 article in the *Journal of Studies on Alcohol* reported that alcohol may interfere with brain development in adolescents, resulting in mild mental impairment. Alcohol-induced changes in the structure or size of the hippocampus (a key part of the brain) may cause lifelong memory problems.

Kids who start drinking young are more likely to have alcohol and other adjustment problems throughout their lives. In 2003 RAND Health, an independent research institute, reported the results of a ten-year study; people who begin to drink by the seventh grade tend to show "employment problems, other substance abuse, and criminal and violent behavior" by age 23.

Of course, some of these people may have underlying problems that led to early drinking *and* later problems. Still, findings like these should make young people sit up and take notice.

WHAT HAPPENS AT 21?

The peak drinking age for Americans is 21. More people drink (67.5 percent in 2001), binge (48.2 percent), and are heavy drinkers (17.8 percent) at age 21 than at any point before or after, according to the 2001 National Household Survey on Drug Abuse. Young people who actually obeyed the laws, and delayed drinking until age 21, may be contributing to these high numbers.

A SERIOUS PROBLEM

More than half of all Americans have their first taste of alcohol before the legal purchasing age of 21. Unfortunately, too many of these under-age drinkers have serious drinking problems. It is no exaggeration to say that underage alcohol abusers may be putting their futures at risk.

See also: Effects on the Body; Law and Drinking, The; Peer Pressure and Alcohol

FURTHER READING

Gail B. Stewart. *Teen Alcoholics*. San Diego, CA: Lucent, 2000.
Michael Windle. *Alcohol Use Among Adolescents*. Thousand Oaks CA: Sage, 1999.

■ VIOLENCE AND ALCOHOL

See: Alcohol and Violence

HOTLINES AND HELP SITES

Alateen
URL: http://www.al-anon.alateen.org/alateen.html
Phone: 1-888-4AL-ANON (8 A.M.–6 P.M. EST, M–F) or check the Web site for contact information in your area
Affiliation: part of Al-Anon, an organization of relatives and friends of alcoholics
Program: regular meetings of young people to discuss their problems and help each other face them
Mission: to help young people deal with problems of alcoholism in their families or among friends. Members meet in small local groups to discuss their problems and provide mutual support

Alcoholics Anonymous
URL: http://www.alcoholics-anonymous.org/index.cfm
Phone: 1-877-934-2522
Program: Worldwide fellowship of men and women from all walks of life who meet together to attain and maintain sobriety.
Mission: To stay sober and help other alcoholics achieve sobriety.

Alcohol Treatment Referral Hotline
Phone: 1-800-ALCOHOL (24 hours a day, 7 days a week)

American Council on Alcoholism
URL: http://www.aca-usa.org/
Phone: 1-800-527-5344 (Alcoholism Treatment HelpLine)

Center for Substance Abuse Treatment

URL: http://findtreatment.samhsa.gov/facilitylocatordoc.htm (helps locate the appropriate treatment facilities in your area)

Phone: 1-800-662-HELP (Referral Helpline, 24 hours a day, 7 days a week)

Affiliation: U.S. Department of Health and Human Services

Mission: to develop and promote better treatment for substance abuse

Freevibe

URL: http://freevibe.com/

Affiliation: National Youth Anti-Drug Media Campaign

Mission: to provide information to young people about alcohol and drugs, and to help kids find alternative interests and activities—"anti-drugs"

Girl Power

URL: http://girlpower.gov/

Affiliation: U.S. Department of Health and Human Services

Mission: to bring health information of all kinds to girls aged 9–13

MADD Youth in Action

URL: http://www.madd.org/madd_programs/0,1056,2044,00.html

Affiliation: Mothers Against Drunk Driving (MADD)

Programs: Students around the country work with adults, with law enforcement officers, or with other students to prevent drunk driving.

National Association for Children of Alcoholics (NACoA) Just for Kids

URL: http://www.nacoa.org/kidspage.htm

Mission: aims to help kids whose parents abuse alcohol

National Council on Alcoholism and Drug Dependence (NCADD)

URL: http://www.ncadd.org/facts/youdir.html

Phone: 1-800-622-2255 (24-hour "hope line" for referral to local groups that can help); or 1-800-654-HOPE (National Intervention Network, to help people who need but do not want help with alcohol problems)

Affiliation: independent nonprofit group founded by alcoholics

Mission: supplies information about all aspects of alcohol and drugs; runs advocacy programs in New York and Washington to help alcoholics and drug addicts and fight addiction

Pages for Kids
URL: http://www.nacoa.org/kidspage.htm
Affiliation: U.S. Department of Health and Human Services
Mission: provide information to kids on all health-related issues; interactive activities and features

Students Examining the Culture of College Drinking
URL: http://findtreatment.samhsa.gov/facilitylocatordoc.htm
Affiliation: National Institute of Alcoholism and Alcohol Abuse
Mission: providing information about alcohol use and abuse for college students; helpful information for all teens, including interactive and multimedia features and additional help sites

GLOSSARY

A.A., or Alcoholics Anonymous the world's first and largest self-help group for alcoholics

abstinence the practice of not drinking any alcoholic beverages

abuse to misuse a substance or to mistreat or cause injury to a person

acetaldehyde a fairly toxic chemical produced by the liver when alcohol is **metabolized**; it can cause numerous unpleasant side effects

acetaminophen a pain-relief and anti-inflammatory drug sold under various brand names such as Tylenol; it can harm the liver if taken together with or right after alcohol

adipose tissue body fat; even moderate drinking can cause a buildup of fat if added to a normal diet

addiction a condition in which a person habitually gives in to a psychological or physical need for a substance such as alcohol, tobacco, or drugs

AIDS acquired immunodeficiency disease; an illness that destroys a person's immune system if left untreated; it is usually transmitted sexually

alcohol expectancy a theory to explain the association of alcohol with violence or sex; people who believe that alcohol all by itself can turn a drinker violent or increase his or her sexual desire may become violent or sexually aggressive when they drink

alcohol psychosis a bout of severe mental illness caused by long-term heavy drinking, often experienced during **withdrawal** and characterized by delusions, violence, convulsions, and other symptoms

alcoholic, alcoholics a person who has a physical and psychological dependence on alcohol

amphetamines a class of mood-changing drugs often used illegally; taken together with alcohol, they can cause severe stomach distress; by keeping drinkers awake, they can lead to dangerous overdoses of alcohol

anorexia nervosa a medical/psychological condition in which the patient is unwilling to eat the minimum amount of food necessary to stay alive and healthy due to the mistaken idea that they are obese; sometimes associated with abuse of alcohol

Antabuse an **aversion drug** widely used to treat alcoholics

antagonist any drug that prevents alcohol from giving the drinker a high

aphrodisiac any food or drink said to increase love or sexual desire

aversion drugs any drug that makes people ill when they drink alcohol, used in treating **alcoholism**

BAC, or blood alcohol count the percentage of alcohol in a fixed volume of blood

BAL, or blood alcohol level the percentage of alcohol in a fixed volume of blood

bootleggers smugglers and wholesale sellers of illegal alcohol during **Prohibition**

bulimia a medical/psychological condition in which the patient subjects his or her body to cycles of binge eating followed by vomiting or other extreme measures to get rid of the excess food; often associated with **alcohol abuse**

chronic long-lasting or repeated, used to describe any illness such as **alcoholism** that is not easily cured

chugging drinking a large quantity of alcohol in as short a time as possible; in other words, drinking faster than the body can process alcohol safely

congeners organic chemicals found in small amounts in alcoholic beverages; they can add flavor, but they also make a hangover worse

conditioning any routine, repeated experience that shapes a person's behavior; for example, people who grow up with parents who drink heavily may be conditioned to consider such behavior normal

counterconditioning any **behavioral therapy** that attempts to **condition** someone to change a behavior that the patient was previously conditioned to adopt

cross-addiction addiction to one drug as a substitute when another drug is unavailable; heroin addicts may be cross-addicted to alcohol

cross-tolerance a tolerance to one drug that makes the user tolerant to other drugs as well, even those he or she has never used

cure a complete recovery from a medical or psychological disease without any risk of its return

date rape forced sexual activity during a voluntary date

delirium tremens (the D.T.'s) intense, terrifying hallucinations that can accompany **withdrawal**, accompanied by high fevers and extremely aggressive behavior

dependence, dependency an intense physical or psychological need for a substance, such as alcohol; without the substance, a dependent person suffers severe discomfort or illness

depressant   a drug that lowers the level of mental and physical activity

detoxification   a course of treatment, usually at a hospital or other facility, aimed at freeing people from alcohol or drug abuse and restoring their bodies to good health

disease theory   the idea that **alcoholism** is a disease rather than a moral failing or a lifestyle choice

disinhibition model   a theory to explain the association of alcohol with violence; alcohol chemically blurs or deadens the parts of the brain that inhibit, or hold back, one's first impulsive reactions

distill   to refine a beverage by heating it and directing the steam into another container where it is condensed back into liquid form

domestic abuse   the repeated mistreatment of a family member or loved one; can be physical, emotional, or sexual

drug interactions   the combined effect on the body that two or more drugs have when used at the same time, for example, alcohol and various prescription drugs

ethanol   the chemical name for drinking alcohol

fermentation   the natural chemical process in which nonalcoholic liquids such as fruit juice or grain mash are turned into alcoholic beverages; the sugar in the mixture turns to alcohol in the presence of yeast

fetal alcohol syndrome (FAS)   a group of birth abnormalities caused by drinking during pregnancy; it can include physical deformities and behavioral problems

gateway drug   the first drug, often alcohol, used by people who later use illegal drugs

hallucination   a sight or sound of something that is not really there

hazing   physical or emotional abuse as part of an initiation process for new members of a college fraternity or other group

histamine   one of the most important **congeners** found in alcoholic beverages

HIV   human immunodeficiency virus, the organism that causes AIDS

hops   a plant added in the brewing process to add flavor, color, and aroma to beer

illicit drugs   drugs that are not legal for consumption, or that are used without a prescription for nonmedical reasons

intoxication   impaired judgment caused by excessive alcohol consumption

kindling   the progressive worsening of symptoms each additional time an alcoholic goes through withdrawal

malting   the first stage in the process of brewing beer, in which grain kernels are allowed to sprout

manic-depressive disorder   also known as bipolar disorder, a brain disorder that causes unusual shifts in a person's mood, energy, and ability to function

marker   a warning sign of a possible serious behavior problem; for example, drinking at a very young age is considered a marker for illegal drug use later

metabolic tolerance   a natural process in which the liver learns to break down, or **metabolize**, a larger amount of a substance, such as alcohol, in a given period of time

metabolism, or metabolize   the process of breaking down a substance in the body, or to break down a substance in the body

methanol   a common **congener** in alcoholic beverages; some believe it is the main cause of a hangover

morality theory   the idea that people become alcoholics through weak morals; it was popular in the eighteenth and nineteenth centuries

Mothers Against Drunk Driving (MADD)   an advocacy group that tries to reduce drunk driving by stronger laws and law enforcement and by information campaigns

Naltrexone   a drug widely used to treat alcoholics

nicotine   the addictive substance found in tobacco

platelet   a type of blood cell that helps heal wounds; heavy drinking may reduce a person's platelet level

progression   movement from one stage of **alcohol dependency** to a more intense, dangerous stage

progressive illness   a condition, such as **alcohol abuse**, that tends to get worse with time

Prohibition   in the United States from 1919 to 1933, the complete ban on the sale or drinking of alcohol

proof   the proportion of alcohol in a given beverage; figured as twice the percentage by volume: a 100 proof beverage is 50 percent alcohol by volume; used in the United States

psychotherapy   a course of treatment, often based on discussion between a patient and a doctor or counselor, aimed at helping patients modify their behaviors and/or improve their mental states

rape   sex without consent, usually by force

recovering alcoholic   according to the disease model of alcoholism, any alcoholic who is currently abstaining or trying to abstain from alcohol

recreational drug   a drug used to get high or change one's mood

resveratrol   a chemical found in red wine that may help prevent aging in moderate drinkers

risk factor   anything, such as family background or personal problems, that might put a person at high risk for alcohol abuse or other dangerous outcome

sexually transmitted disease (STD) any disease that can be passed from one person to another during sexual relations

sobriety abstaining from alcohol (or other addictive drug)

social drinking moderate drinking in a social context

speakeasy illegal bar in the **Prohibition** era

stepping stone a drug whose users will often move on to another, more dangerous drug, according to some researchers; for example, alcohol is considered by some to be a stepping stone to marijuana

stimulant a drug that makes you feel wide-awake and full of energy

substance abuse any unhealthy or unsafe use of alcohol, illegal drugs, prescription drugs, or any other chemical

syndrome any collection of unhealthy symptoms or behaviors that usually appear together

tagging the practice of marking beer kegs by the seller so that kegs found at parties of underage students can be traced back to the source

temperance movement a movement that arose in England and the United States in the eighteenth century to advocate moderation in drinking; eventually, some temperance supporters became advocates of **prohibition**

tolerance the state in which the body has become accustomed to alcohol or another substance, so that a person needs to drink more to get the same mental effect

toxic poisonous

tremors shaking

twelve-step program any treatment program for alcoholism or other addiction that stresses the Twelve Steps to recovery developed by A.A. (Alcoholics Anonymous)

tyramine   a chemical found naturally in beer and red wine, that can dangerously increase blood pressure if a drinker also uses MAOI antidepressants

venereal disease   former term for **sexually transmitted disease**

Volstead Act   the 1919 law that put **Prohibition** into effect in the United States

withdrawal   the combination of painful and uncomfortable symptoms alcoholics feel when they stop or drastically cut back their drinking

zero tolerance   a policy of enforcing and prosecuting even the most minor incidence of any law, such as drunk-driving or drug-possession laws

INDEX

Page numbers in *italic* indicate graphs or sidebars. Page numbers in **bold** represent extensive coverage of a topic.